SOMETHING NOT QUITE RIGHT

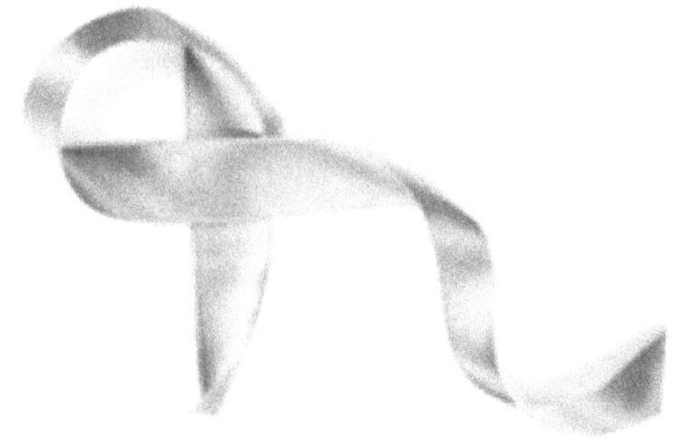

**A GRIPPING TRUE STORY
OF DEALING WITH
MENTAL ILLNESS
AND GOD'S HEALING**

LUKE & JENNY ZIMMERMANN

Table of Contents

Prologue

Mental illness snuck up on us and it took years to realize what we were dealing with.

Here are some data: according to the Australian Institute of Health and Welfare (2019), 45% of the population between 16 and 85 years old, or 7.3 million people, suffered from a mental disorder at some point in their life. This echoes the exact number stated by Australian Bureau of Statistics 12 years earlier (2007). The ABS National Survey of Health and Well-being in 2008 found that "the proportion of Australians estimated to have a long-term mental or behavioral problem increased progressively between 1995 and 2005." The Mental Health Foundation in the UK reports that 1 in 4 people will experience some kind of mental health problem in the course of a year. The use of anti-depressants is constantly on the rise and the number of people taking them now runs in the many hundreds of millions. According to the National Institute of Mental Health, one in 17 Americans suffers from serious mental illness. Although reliable figures of other countries are hard to obtain, there is no reason to assume that the situation is any different there.

It is also a misconception that depression will not affect Christians. Unfortunately many Christians feel it is unspiritual to feel depressed or anxious and shows a lack of faith. it may even be seen as sinful and therefore rather not acknowledge. (Tan & Ortberg, 2004).

Jenny and I wrote this book because we have a story to tell. It is our sincere desire that our story will help those who are in the same situation as us: confused by mental illness, overwhelmed by its complications and its wide variety of manifestations. Above all, this story was written to encourage and give hope to Christians and non-Christians alike: there are answers, there are solutions, there is healing. Our story describes these.

I am writing because others have written their stories before me and have encouraged me in my darkest moments, at times when I had lost all hope and could not see anything remotely positive in my life and my future.

For at least 25 years, I've been indirectly affected by mental illness. Here's a summary: I've worked for three mentally ill bosses – one alcoholic and two schizophrenics. At the same time, my wife, Jenny, suffered from severe depression and eventually developed schizophrenia. About ten years later, our son, Mitchel, started suffering from depression at the age of 15 and turned bi-polar within the next year and a half. Finally, and I pray that this is finally, our daughter, Chantelle, became clinically depressed and has just developed a less severe form of bi-polar disorder. This book does not cover their story. Others in the family and in our constantly changing circle of friends (who don't want to be mentioned) suffered from different forms of mental illness; some with dire consequences. Although I became depressed myself and had a short time on an anti-depressant, I am writing from a carer's perspective.

My wife, Jenny, tells her side of the story (in a different font). If you have to deal with mental illness, her experience will deeply touch you.

Not one of the incidents and events described in this book is fiction. Every detail of this story is as close to reality as words would allow. Only the names of the people outside our family have been changed to conceal their identity.

Dedication and thanks

This book is obviously dedicated to Jesus, our Lord and Saviour. Without Him, this story would never have been written because it would not have had a good ending. He is "the healer of our heart and the lover of our soul" and without Him we would have given up years ago.

The Lord put some of His faithful people around us to counsel us and help us. We will forever be grateful to Evelyn Swain who patiently counselled Jenny for many months and Jean Tivinan who provided us so generously with all kinds of practical help. Also many thanks to Glenn and Noreen O'Brien and Guy and Debbie Ormerod who were great role models for Jenny and me when we met weekly in their home.

We also want to dedicate this book to the psychiatrists who have helped us beyond the call of duty. They advised us with endless patience and compassion: on the Gold Coast in Australia Dr Finnemore at the hospital and in the United Arab Emirates Dr Talaat in Ras Al Khaimah.

Finally, we dedicate this book to those who suffer from mental illness and those who care for them. May our story encourage you and give you hope.

God bless you.

Luke and Jenny Zimmermann

CHAPTER 1 The train to Paris

Amsterdam, The Netherlands, 1980

It was six in the morning and not my favourite time to be awake. I was mighty glad I had made it to Central Station and plonked down in a seat in the train carriage that was going to take me to Paris. In Rotterdam, my friend Tom would join me and the plan was to hitch-hike from Paris to the Dordogne in the south-east of France to do some work on my dad's holiday house. After a whole night's party and I don't know how many beers, I had arrived home at four in the morning and for two hours desperately tried not to fall asleep. I had cycled to Central station and I still felt quite drunk. Now I had made it to the train, I started to relax. I could go to sleep and if I didn't wake up in Rotterdam, I was sure Tom would find me.

Behind me, some people spoke in German. It jolted me because I thought I was in the wrong train. I had noticed that there were two trains waiting back-to-back on the platform. One had a sign that said Frankfurt, Germany on it and the other one Paris, France. Was I in the wrong train? I knew I was in the last carriage but had I stepped onto the German train in my drunken state? I better get up and check. With difficulty, I got out of the comfortable seat. Grabbing my bag, I stumbled out of the carriage back onto the platform. I checked the sign, Paris, France. Still swaying a bit, my legs somewhat wobbly, a female voice from behind me drifted into my foggy brain:

"Excuse me, is this the train to Paris?" I said: "I think so" and turned around. A young lady, probably my age, very well-dressed, long blond hair and make-up on, approached me. It struck how very fresh she looked compared to me after an all-nighter and no shower for more than a few days. I suddenly felt unclean, something that never normally bothered me. As a student living in a room on the fourth floor with no bathroom, hygiene was not high on my list of priorities.

"Are you going to Paris?"

"Yes, I am." she said with enthusiasm.

"Where are you from?" I asked because I didn't recognise her accent straightaway. I could hear she was not British and not American and obviously not Dutch, since she started the conversation in English. But it wasn't clear to me where she was from.

"I'm Australian."

She stepped into the carriage and started walking along the aisle to find a place. Following her, I was wondering whether I should sit next to her. Would that be too pushy? She didn't really look like my type anyway, way too sophisticated and not like the unkempt female university students I was used to in Amsterdam. Then I heard a clear voice in my head saying:

"You are going to Australia with this woman."

It was almost audible and I looked around to see if anyone else had heard it but no one looked surprised. The girl suddenly turned around, stuck out her hand and said:

"My name is Jenny Penning."

We shook hands and I introduced myself.

"Are you from here?"

"Yes, I am Dutch and I live here in Amsterdam. I am a student."

The conversation had started and it was easy to continue. It probably would have been rude not to sit next to her: "Do you mind?"

Tom joined us in Rotterdam and we talked for five hours, mostly in Dutch, because Jenny said she wanted to learn the language. It was years afterwards when she told me she had only understood about 10 percent of the conversation but was just happy to be laughing with us. We were joking about Australia, the funny accent, the lack of culture, as we haughty Europeans perceived it, and, of course, the kangaroos.

When we arrived in Paris, we said goodbye. She was hoping for an invitation to join us but I never asked her. I thought it would be too difficult to hitch-hike with three people and I wasn't really sure how I felt about this girl yet. It was clear she was not my type, not intellectual enough, and I couldn't imagine she would be interested in me. I also thought that she would most probably like Tom more than me because that is what usually happened with girls we met. They would usually fall for Tom. He was a bit shorter than me and much better built. He had blond hair and blue eyes and was a very sensitive guy. I felt somewhat inferior next to him, since I was 6 foot 5 and very skinny. My dark hair and greenish eyes were also nothing special. On top of that, I was normally very shy, except when I had a reasonable amount of alcohol in me.

The only thing I thought was in my favour was that Jenny also lived in Amsterdam and I invited her to a party at my house when I returned in two weeks. When we said goodbye she looked lost and sad but, as a fairly self-centered, fiercely independent Dutchman, I had no time to worry about that because we had a long way to go and first had to find our way out of Paris.

When we were working in my dad's house, I slowly started to realize that I was falling in love. There was a pop song playing on the radio in Holland called 'Falling in love with Jenny' and although I couldn't stand the song, it kept coming up in my mind and I found myself singing it aloud while I was working. Tom caught me a number of times and thought it was hilarious. He told me he had no interest in the girl and I was surprised to feel a great relief. This was all very strange. How could I be interested in a girl who was not a student and was not a rational, analytical thinker? My head and my heart gave me completely opposite signals. It was confusing but, in the end, I just decided to enjoy the feeling of falling in love because it had been a long time and I thought I'd sort it out when I'd meet her again. I had forgotten about the voice in my head.

When I picked Jenny up for the party two weeks later, I was extremely nervous. By then she had become a fascinating, highly intelligent super-woman in my mind and I felt some nagging concern that the picture in my mind was utter fantasy and that she would be a great disappointment. In addition, I was worried that I would not fit her expectations of a boy-friend. I had no experience with this kind of women or Australians for that matter. The only thing that gave me some confidence was the fact that she had laughed a lot at my jokes. I knocked on the door of the small apartment on the third floor where she was staying with her aunt and uncle. After quick introductions, we left. She still looked very fresh to me and I was glad I had had a shower and a shave and looked more presentable this time. It struck me that night that she was certainly not the superwoman of my imagination, but she was very down-to-earth and uncomplicated. However, this was surprisingly refreshing. It was also obvious that she was a pretty quiet person and the conversation was somewhat one-sided. After a few beers, it was always easier for me to talk, but I had decided not to get drunk. I didn't want her to think that that is how I usually was and that I could only function socially with alcohol in me.

The silence was somewhat awkward at times and I left her a few times on her own pretending to have to attend to something to keep the party going. I still wasn't sure what I was doing with her, but there was some strange attraction, in a way I had never experienced before. Her simplicity and unpretentious attitude were disarming and even quite sexy. All previous girlfriends had been intellectuals, usually strongly independent, and I had always built friendships with girls first before falling in love. The intellectual discussions would turn me on and suddenly I'd see beauty in women that I didn't find attractive at first sight.

With Jenny, everything was different. She had a certain soft melancholic expression on her face and gorgeous blue eyes. I also noticed that she had quite a good figure. She reached to my shoulder and half-way through the evening I bent over and I gave her a quick kiss. There was no resistance at all and when I took her home in my old car, I kissed her again. She turned to me and kissed me back so openly, it disarmed me completely. She even put her right hand on the back of my neck and gently touched my cheek. Maybe I had expected her to be quite shy about physical contact but she seemed utterly relaxed. It felt really good and we melted into each others' arms. Unfortunately my car was not the most comfortable place for an embrace and soon my back started to twitch. Since there was nowhere else to go, I gently let go and suggested we would part now and see each other the next day. I didn't want to push this relationship too quickly anyway because I had a feeling that this was going to be unusual and I wanted to savor every moment. I walked her to the front door, arms around each other, and kissed her goodbye. I drove home singing at the top of my voice.

In the following few weeks, we saw each other almost every day. We went for long walks in different places and talked. She told me about her life and family in Australia and I told her about my life. We were both surprised that we got on so well because we were so different. We had very different backgrounds and were used to very different kinds of friends. I was an academic who loved studying and discussing issues, whereas Jenny was from a working class family, had left school at fifteen and had worked ever since. At the age of twenty-three, she had decided to leave Australia and fly to Holland to see where her parents had come from. They were originally Dutch and had migrated to Australia in the early fifties.

In Sydney, Jenny had friends who were much older than her. She was used to going out with guys who were in their late twenties or early thirties and found people of her own age in Australia too immature. She was surprised at the depth of conversation she could have with me. She was also surprised at the fact that I was not in a hurry to sleep with her; guys in Australia were always in a rush, she said.

We really enjoyed each others' company in those few weeks, but the bad news was that I had to go to the UK for the next seven weeks. I was booked into a study program with the Wycliffe Bible Translators to learn about field-linguistics. I considered canceling the course but it had taken a friend of mine and me a long time to convince our professor at the University of Amsterdam that this was a good course and would complement our linguistics master's degree. Jenny became very quiet and gloomy when I told her this. To my surprise, I couldn't stand the idea that I wouldn't see her for all that time, so I suggested she would come to England to visit me. She was keen. She would take a week or two off and come to the UK. This was perfect as she had come to Holland to travel around Europe anyway.

A few weeks later I was in High Wycombe, halfway between London and Oxford.

It was a quiet, little town in the hills and the slopes were full of wild flowers at this time of year. The course was run in an old army camp and the accommodation was fairly simple. It was not my idea of a good time to be in the middle of a camp, full of Christians who were eager to learn about linguistics and foreign languages so they could be sent out as missionaries and translate the Bible. At the time I was not a Christian. In fact, I was extremely anti-Christian and I considered myself an atheist. There was quite a mix of people in the group – from very pleasant and accepting to very pushy Bible bashers. My friend and I were told that we had not really been alive, because we didn't know Christ. That didn't make any sense to me. At night, we escaped to the Studley Arms, a beautiful, old English pub which happened to be right opposite the army camp.

When Jenny arrived, I was settled into a routine of study and other camp duties. It had seemed like an eternity as I had really missed her. We found a nice bed-and-breakfast in town and stayed there for a week. Every morning we had English breakfasts in the dining room with a view over the beautiful hills. One morning the landlady knocked on our door early and urged us to come and have breakfast. When we asked why, we were told that Prince Charles and Diana were going to be married that day and that she really didn't want to miss a minute of it. Neither of us could relate to the excitement. We had no interest whatsoever in the British royal family. We went out that day to explore the surroundings and ended up sitting on a hillside in a most beautiful spot in the afternoon sun. The view was stunning – rolling hills full of colored flowers waving in a gentle breeze. I was sitting behind Jenny and put my arms around her. I was happy to just sit there quietly and enjoy the memory of a perfect day together, when I noticed that she had a very sad expression on her face. "What's the matter?"

She said that she suddenly felt really low for no reason. She probably missed her family. I couldn't really understand this. First of all, why would you miss your family? And secondly, how could you feel low, while you were in such a beautiful place and after such a great day together? Did she have enough of me? Did she suddenly realise it wasn't going to work for her? I was bewildered for the first time.

The next day Jenny was her normal cheerful self and we didn't discuss what had happened the previous day. We had a great week together and had become best friends and lovers. At the end of the week we unfortunately had to say goodbye as she returned to Holland, back to work. She left a great void. We wrote each other almost every day with the letters becoming more and more intense. We missed each other so much and poured our hearts out on page after and page of increasingly emotional language. It was hard to focus on my study. An endless five weeks later, I finally went back home myself with a stack of love letters. Lying on the deck of the ferry over the English Channel, soaking up the sun, I felt tremendously relieved to be out of the army camp and away from those Christians. I just couldn't understand them and their beliefs. I would have laughed if someone had told me then that I was going to be a born-again Christian myself one day.

When I arrived in Amsterdam, I went straight to Jenny's house. I was so looking forward to seeing her again. She had been this completely new breeze in my life because she was different from any person I had ever met and I was now really in love with her. We had really missed each other and had been very frank about it in our writing. She had also changed her accommodation. When government housing is being renovated, the city of Amsterdam provides the local residents with temporary accommodation in the form of relocatable cabins. A friend of the family had found some empty ones that were no longer in use. It was common in those days to just break into one of these cabins, claim it as your new home and rock up at the Department of Housing to pay a nominal rent. So they did. These cabins were fitted out with all the comforts – a bathroom, kitchen and two small bedrooms. It also had a big gas heater in it. It was luxury compared to my student room.

When I knocked on the door, I expected Jenny to be extremely happy to see me. Instead, she seemed depressed and distant. She had been expecting me much earlier in the day and had been waiting for hours and hours. It took some time to reconnect with her, but soon we were back where we had left off in the UK.

The next year and a half Jenny and I became inseparable. I couldn't stand being away from her for more than one day. There was such a strong pull to be together and we had both accepted that we were supposed to be together despite our big differences in personality and background. We went on holidays together and we decided she would give up her cabin to save the rent money. Although we didn't discuss it, we both knew that she would have to move in with me when we returned from the holidays. And so we started living together.

My room was quite large for Dutch standards, but had only one tiny window that looked out onto De Lairessestraat, a main street through the old southern part of Amsterdam. One day I found Jenny standing quietly staring out of the window. I asked if she was ok. Without turning to me, she asked

"How can you live in this place?"

I didn't understand the question. I had lived in many rooms in Amsterdam and this was the best one. It was spacious and it had some nice antique furniture in it. I had some good friends living on the same floor and the floor beneath, so I was very happy there and, in fact, quite proud of my abode.

"What do you mean?"

"Look! There is hardly any light. When you look outside, you only see multi-story houses and no blue sky. It's so depressing. Come and look."

I walked over to the window and although I was looking at the same view as her, I could not see what she saw. She told me about the vast blue skies in Australia and the endless sunshine, the outdoor life and the enormous space in this almost empty country.

Jenny grew more and more restless in Amsterdam and became homesick. We decided she would go back to Australia for a short time. I was hoping that she just needed to see her family and old friends, realize that nothing had changed there and she would come back to Holland with her mind at ease. She agreed and organized her flight back. I had no money to join her at that time and was still very busy with my study and a part-time job I had. So Jenny left and I was on my own again. I wasn't sure whether I was going to see her again.

A week later, my neighbour from downstairs woke me up at 2.30 in the morning. "Jenny is on the phone."

I ran downstairs and still half asleep picked up the receiver.

"Do you still love me?"

"What? Are you ringing me in the middle of the night for this?"

"Yes, sorry, but I need to know now."

Her voice sounded urgent and nervous.

"Yes, I do," I said not too convincingly. I wasn't sure whether this was real or whether I was dreaming.

"Why do you need to know that now? What's going on?"

She told me that she had met her old boyfriend in Australia and he had asked her to marry him. He had never stopped loving her and wanted to settle down with her. I gathered from the conversation that he was in many respects the opposite of me - he was about 10 years older, was a psychologist and had a Porsche. I asked her what she wanted to do. I was not the type to push her in any direction. I strongly believed that people should be free to make their own choices and if she felt strongly about it, it was up to her.

"I don't know. I need to know that you love me and you want me to come back."

I hated this situation. I didn't want to make a decision for her, because I was not a hundred percent clear about my own feelings. My mind was frantic. I wasn't even properly awake and I had to make a major decision about my life. What to do? We talked for a while longer and my mind flashed to the future – a future without Jenny. Imagine I would never see her again and I would not know what would happen to her. I would never kiss her again, hold her in my arms and smell her hair. It looked empty and dreary. I told her that I wanted her to come back. She sounded relieved and, before she hung up the phone, she promised to book a flight back as soon as possible.

When we met at the airport, Jenny looked quite different. She had lost many kilos and looked quite skinny. She had tears in her eyes when she saw me. We touched hands through the glass and, when she came through the gate, we hugged for a long time. She told me she always stopped eating when she was nervous.

"You were right. Nothing had changed in Australia and although it was good to see everyone, I wanted to come back here. And by the way, they didn't like my new spiky hairstyle at all. They were shocked to see me like that."

In the following months we grew closer and started talking seriously about migrating to Australia.

The summer was approaching and we started to plan a trip. Jen wanted to see Europe and I suggested cycling. It took a bit of convincing her but we finally decided to buy bicycles, put them on the train to Vienna and follow the river Danube through Hungary into Yugoslavia. After that, we would take the train to Istanbul and cycle into Turkey. That holiday everything went according to plan and we were having the time of our lives. Riding a bike everyday made us fit and strong and many people approached us in a very positive way. With all the sunshine Jenny's hair became blonder and her skin bronzed. Many times I looked at her during those weeks and considered myself so lucky that a beautiful woman like her would even be interested in me. I fell madly in love with her. When we arrived in Istanbul, I wasn't the only one looking. Istanbul was a male-dominated city in the early 80s. In fact, we didn't see any women on the streets at all. We were walking around in shorts and Jen was wearing a tight, open top. This attracted way too much attention for my liking. At some stage I looked around and saw about a hundred heads turned eying Jenny. It all of a sudden hit me how naïve it was to walk around in a Muslim country with a beautiful blonde woman in shorts. I gently pulled Jen to the side and said:

"We're going to get you some clothes."

We bought some long pants and a top that covered her figure a little and we continued exploring the city. After six weeks we arrived back in Amsterdam and started thinking about leaving Holland for good.

After numerous phone calls and letters with Australia House in The Hague that authorizes all immigration to Australia, it was clear that the only way I was going to get a permanent resident visa was if we got married. This was not an easy decision, of course. Neither of us was in a hurry to get married and we both still felt a bit young at 24 for such a major commitment. My proposal was decidedly unromantic:

"So shall we get married then?"

"Yeah?"

"Well, if you want to go back to Australia and I want to go there too, and we want to stay together, then we have no choice. We want to stay together, right?"

"Yes, we do. We can always try and if it doesn't work out in the end, we can go our own way."

So it was decided. We put in all the paperwork to Australia House and waited. We wanted to have our wedding in Australia on a beach with a marriage celebrant. This was explained to Australia House in a letter and we had asked for confirmation that this was acceptable. We heard nothing. When the airplane tickets arrived, I decided to contact Australia House to make sure all was well. They checked our file and told me that we needed a letter from a celebrant stating the date and place of the wedding. We didn't know any celebrants and we only had six weeks before we were due to fly out. What now? It all seemed so rushed. We rang the marriage registry. There was only one space available on the twenty-first of December. We booked it. We didn't want a big wedding; we just needed the piece of paper to get a visa.

On the twenty-first of December 1982, I dressed up in my best clothes and Jenny in her new winter dress and we left for our wedding on my old black hallelujah bicycle. As always, Jenny hopped on the back. We had thick coats on because it was cold outside. Fortunately, it wasn't raining. I cycled through the Vondel Park and then into the inner city along its beautiful canals. The trip to the registry office was not at all how we had ever imagined to get married but we both thought it was very romantic and enjoyed the fact that it was so unconventional. We laughed a lot along the way, feeling ecstatic.

We met our two witnesses, Tom and Jenny's friend who helped her squat the cabin, in front of the building, took some photos and went in. We were married in a very simple ceremony by a black lady and signed the papers. Straight after we left for The Hague to hand in our marriage certificate to Australia House. It took them less than five minutes to hand me my passport with my resident visa. I couldn't believe it. We celebrated with a few drinks and a meal with Tom and his girlfriend in Rotterdam.

Four weeks later, I said goodbye to my family and friends and we left for Australia.

CHAPTER 2 A Gift from God

Fairfield, Western Sydney, Australia 1988

When our son Mitchel was born in Fairfield Hospital at midday on the eighth of October 1988, God put a big rainbow in the sky to celebrate his arrival. Jenny had been convinced that it was going to be a girl and we were so relieved when the labor was finally over that we wrapped our new-born up in a towel and didn't even check the gender until we heard the nurse ask:

"Is it a boy or a girl?"

I liked the fact that she didn't just tell us. I am sure she would have noticed. I unwrapped the baby and my eyes popped wide open:

"It's a boy!"

We were so surprised that it was a boy that we didn't actually have a name for him. Within the hour, Jenny's mum arrived and said that she had actually got a few male names prepared just in case.

"What about Mitchel or......."

Nobody seemed to hear the other names because we all liked Mitchel straightaway. The nurse, who only heard part of the conversation, immediately wrote the name 'Mitchel' on the card and we were too tired to protest. The name stuck and was never changed. Later we found out that Mitchel meant 'gift from God', a name we really liked.

Our son was not an easy baby. He was very restless and kept us up at night in an almost regular pattern: he'd sleep for one hour and then he'd be up crying for an hour and a half. In that time he was breastfed and his nappy changed. We then spent up to an hour calming him down by rubbing him on his back. He usually and finally settled down after a big burp. It was an exhausting routine and since I always tried to be the supportive husband, Jenny and I did this together. One day we took Mitchel to the doctor after he had been up for three nights in a row. He just wouldn't settle down and we were exasperated. At the baby clinic, we saw a young doctor and explained the problem. He looked at us with a smirk on his face and said:

"Your first one, is it?"

His patronizing tone infuriated me but I said nothing. I was too worn-out to respond. We ended up going home with no solution, only some useless advice like "try to relax". In the meantime, I was working full-time as a teacher and after six weeks of sleepless nights, I broke. I was standing in the kitchen and was about to cook some dinner, when I just started crying. I was so exhausted, I couldn't go on. Jenny let me sleep through the night that night and I felt like a different person the next day. It wasn't until a year later that we learnt about colic and realized that Mitchel had been suffering from severe colic.

I was so supportive that I was doing the washing, cleaning, cooking and anything else that had to be done. Jenny did some shopping, but spent most of her time in the rocking chair holding Mitchel. They would listen to Hare Krishna chanting all day long. It was one of the only things that would settle Mitchel down.

For the last six years Jenny and I had been delving into spiritual matters. We had started with meditation, then Buddhism, Hinduism and were now deeply involved with a famous Indian guru. Even Time magazine featured an article about him with the title "God on earth". I was convinced he was, because he performed so many miracles and if someone had that much power, he must be from God. Through meditation, I had become calm and peaceful inside and felt much happier than I had ever felt before. Because of this, we had expected our son to be peaceful too. Nothing was further from the truth and he became a great concern to us and was Jenny's main focus during the day and mine at night.

We were up at five every morning, when Mitchel was ready to start the day. Jenny would do washing and hang it out while I spent time with Mitch, make breakfast and lunch and get ready for work. I had to take the train to the center of Sydney, which took about an hour door-to-door. When I came home from work, I'd take the washing off the line and fold it, spend some time with Jen and Mitch and start cooking. Every day was different. One day Jenny would clean and tidy, the next she wouldn't do anything because she'd be totally absorbed in her own thoughts. After dinner, I'd wash up and did other chores that needed to be done. It did occur to me that Jenny was not doing very much, but she told me that she was so tired all the time and that Mitchel needed so much attention. It seemed to me that Jenny was not enjoying being a mum and she didn't look good, almost as if she had never recovered from giving birth. She didn't look after herself and didn't seem to care what she was wearing anymore. She had lost a lot of weight and was quite skinny again. Socializing became a chore for her, too. She was no longer involved in the conversations and withdrew more and more. She often had excuses for not wanting to meet people and even for not wanting to do anything. The excuses were usually very "spiritual".

I truly loved being a Mum but, indeed, I wasn't enjoying it the way that I had imagined I would. I was very busy just coping with how I was feeling and this took up the better part of the day.

The birth had been tough. The labor and the contractions were excruciatingly painful and I realized with intense knowingness that I didn't want to do this. I was afraid, so terribly afraid, and suddenly, for the first time in my life, I couldn't stop it, control it or make it go away. I wanted so desperately to have a baby and yet I was scared beyond belief.

The gas was good and I even had to fight Luke for the mask once. He was going through his own feelings of anxiety and helplessness. We had had breathing classes but now it was the real thing and I wasn't coping. In desperation Luke yelled "scream!" and I did. Finally I felt relief, so I screamed and screamed and couldn't stop screaming. It felt so good. I had an intense feeling of well-being and power. I felt like I had conquered the world. Years later I realized that the screaming had broken through the boundaries in my mind that had been in place all my life. They were now gone. On the one hand, this had been a very liberating experience and made me feel incredibly powerful; yet on the other hand, it made me feel extremely helpless.

Our son was born and, with his eyes wide open, he checked out the entire room and the people in it. Initially, when I arrived home from the hospital, I had constant diarrhea. For days on end I was walking around with a towel between my legs in case of any accidents. It wasn't until my sister-in-law suggested something from the pharmacy that I realized that I was living in my own little world and wasn't coping at all well.

A lot of the time when I wasn't busy with Mitchel, I was in a trance of sorts. I would sit in the rocking chair looking at the wall in front of me. I suddenly became aware of choirs of angels; they were so beautiful and then along with them came visions of the end of the world graphically displayed. The sight of all the fire and brimstone I imagined would be very scary; however, for some reason unbeknownst to me I was in fact totally detached from it all. The scenes were so real that I felt I could reach out and touch them. Why I saw this and for what purpose, I had no idea at all.

These visions had started when I was pregnant with Mitchel and still working. As with most pregnant women in the late stage of pregnancy, the need to pee had become increasingly persistent. One day I went to the toilet and as always I took the first cubical. Whilst relieving myself, I became fixated on a spot on the marble door in front of me. Suddenly I felt my hand stretch out and the marble door turn to jelly. I stuck my hand right into the door. Just then someone came in, I pulled my hand back and my train of thought and focus was gone.

As a new mum, I was always looking for ways to keep Mitchel happy and content. Apart from listening to chanting and classical music, rocking in the rocking chair and rides in the car, we went for long walks while he slept in the baby pouch against my chest. On these walks I would spend my time thinking about many different new age concepts and how to continue with my personal development. I really hungered for more self-awareness, especially now that I was seeing all these things that I had no way of understanding at all. I became progressively self-absorbed. I truly believed that God had chosen me to do some kind of major deed for him. All the while Mitchel would receive great care not only because I loved him so much but also because I believed he was indeed a wonderful gift from God and was also destined to do great things.

While walking I would think about some of the self-help courses we had done. One in particular was about reflection. In the course we were told that what you see in others is what you are yourself. I took it one step further. I argued with myself that if we were reflections of each other then we were also reflections of the beauty around us. From here I began to believe that everything I looked at was a reflection of myself. Whether it was beautiful or ugly, however I perceived it, that was me. This was the real beginning of my confusion.

Slowly but surely every day I began to see more intricate patterns of the capacity of what my brain could do. It went on and on until one day I realized that I could actually see things before they happened. That's when it got really scary. I began to see lots of different things happen which were not good. There were car accidents, dogs and cats being run over by cars, and on and on. From that point on, life became unbearable. I realized that because in the new age we were taught that we create our own reality I began to believe that I was creating all of this mayhem and the fact that it wouldn't stop happening meant that I must have been very bad. I was constantly feeling guilty about every single detail of life. If I saw it then I must have created it.

My whole life I had been good and now it seemed I had become the opposite and felt incredibly tormented by this burden. I saw earthquakes in the future and thought that I must have created them. A simple newspaper report of an earthquake having occurred would make me cringe and sink within myself, feeling responsible. The whole world was on my shoulders and I began to be afraid. I thought I must be going mad. Yet I would not go to a doctor in case they locked me up.

I lost the ability to cook. Knowing the difference between rice and vegetables and how long they each took to cook was beyond me. But thank God I had Luke. He took over. He went to work by day and when he got home, he did what I couldn't do. He stayed by my side and supported me through severe post-natal depression. We didn't know this at the time. I could simply have gotten medical help and all would have been well but I was afraid that I would be committed to the "nuthouse" and so I didn't go to a doctor but chose to go through it totally on my own.

All of this made me incredibly protective of our son. I saw to his every need and became totally engrossed in care, play and nurturing him as a mother.

At work things were intense and stressful. I was working as an English language teacher in a Japanese owned college. It was a place where foreign students came to study English from anything between two weeks and one year. The business was booming especially after the Australian government agreed to issue student visas to the Chinese. I was promoted to program coordinator which involved supervising language programs and staff. The owner and managing director, Mr Jay Honda, was thrilled of course. His secretaries were counting enrolment fees in the form of cheques and cash for hours every day. Literally millions of dollars were pouring in. However, Mr Honda had never been a good communicator and was, like most Japanese, extremely self-conscious about speaking English, especially in front of his senior staff. The fact that we were all English language teachers made it even more stressful. Every time he joined us in a meeting, which was not very often at all, he seemed very nervous and some of us noticed alcohol on his breath. One day, he walked into a coordinators' meeting and said in a strong Japanese accent: "In sree mons, twelve hundred Chinese students come. Organize it!" and walked out. We were stunned and first had to check with each other whether we had understood correctly what he had said. Was he for real? Twelve hundred Chinese? Couldn't he give us some more detail and direction? What was wrong with him?

Somehow we managed to organize the programs and the college grew from one hundred and fifty students to fifteen hundred in the next three months. Most of these Chinese spoke no English at all and we were all on a steep learning curve to try and cope with this influx. In the meantime, the more money Mr Honda made the weirder his behavior became. During the Christmas party at the Hilton hotel, he gave a speech. He thanked us all for our hard work and gave us some information about the company. It was hard to focus on his words because he had a piece of bread in his hands which he was pulling apart; he stuffed little pieces of bread in his mouth and slowly chewed on it while he continued to speak. It seemed to me that he was quite unaware of what he was doing and I felt sorry for him. On the other hand, it was hard not to laugh. It wasn't until years later that I wondered if he was suffering from some kind of mental illness.

Mr Honda became quite abusive when the smallest thing went wrong. He would call individual teachers into his office and give them what we started to call 'a Japanese treatment', which usually ended up in yelling. All this created an enormous amount of stress among the staff. One day I got my turn. He took me into a classroom and asked me to open the cupboard. There were a few books in there that belonged to the college. In a patronizing tone of voice, he told me to read the stamp on the cover and then lectured me for ten minutes on the cost of these books and that I should make sure they were not left lying around the college. The fact that the cupboard was locked was dismissed as irrelevant. The whole discussion was quite bizarre and I decided to just let him rave on until he was finished. That took about forty minutes. After half an hour I went quiet and eventually Mr Honda ran out of things to say. I left the classroom furious about the treatment I had received but there was nothing I could do.

Mr Honda started to drink more and more. One day a television crew arrived at the college to interview him about the growth in the industry but he was nowhere to be found. His secretary, with the film crew in-tow, walked all around the college and checked all the rooms. The camera was rolling. They finally found Mr Honda deep asleep with an empty whiskey bottle next to the bed in the sick room. It was ten in the morning and this was not good news for the business. The rumor was that it took some fast talking by the general manager and a substantial amount of money to keep this story from going to air.

It was an exciting time, too. I had a new job and learnt a lot of new skills. I had to learn computer programs, manage teaching staff and run meetings. I spent a lot of time working through my shyness and forced myself to participate in meetings. As a non-native speaker, I was also self-conscious about speaking English in front of the teaching staff but I had no choice. I started with small irrelevant comments like

"Can I open the window? It's hot in here"

and slowly built up to longer and more relevant contributions to the meetings. It was a liberating process.

After four years in this job, Jenny and I decided we needed a change. I was sick of the rat race and wanted an alternative lifestyle. We were going to move up north, to the country, buy a house and start a business. This was a dream we had had since we left Holland. The Australian government had stopped issuing Chinese student visas after the slaughter at Tiananmen Square in June 1989. Colleges all around Sydney were closing down and numerous teachers were laid off. Our college was also shrinking rapidly. I had a choice: if I became a union member, I could stay in my job but would be demoted to teaching. If I did not join the teachers' union, I would be laid off and receive a redundancy payment. I choose the latter and left the college exactly two weeks before we had to vacate our house. We had sold our house and put all our possessions in storage and would have it transported to our new location, eight hundred kilometers north of Sydney, as soon as we had found a place to live.

Two months later, I received a letter from my old colleagues that the college had closed down unexpectedly. Teachers arrived for work one day to find the doors permanently closed. Mr Honda had disappeared. It was a carefully orchestrated scam. The day before the college closed, the secretary was still taking money from students who wanted to extend their courses or enroll for the first time. Most of the money was transferred into a Swiss bank account and Mr Honda had fled the country. All staff were owed salaries. I felt incredibly lucky I had taken the redundancy package.

CHAPTER 3 Hippie time
Nimbin, Northern NSW, Australia, 1990

The northern part of New South Wales is gorgeous. It is hilly and green and around every bend in the road is another stunning view. Jenny and I fell in love with the area when we visited it a year earlier and decided that if we had the chance we would move here. When we drove into Nimbin, an isolated village deep into this hilly country, it felt like we were coming home. Here time had stood still since the 1970s when the hippies had congregated here for a large festival. Many of them never left and built humpies in the bush in an attempt to go back to nature. In 1990 there were still many hippies in town – long hair, flowery dresses and little kids with bare bottoms everywhere. There was a large health food store in town that sold tofu and other vegetarian food and a greengrocery that specialized in organically grown fruit and vegetables. Since we had become vegetarians, this was a very attractive place to settle down.

We bought a piece of land in a new subdivision, a few minutes' drive out of town, and bought an old house from Brisbane – about three hours' drive north of Nimbin. The house was delivered in two halves on huge trucks and put together again when it was positioned on our land. I renovated the house over the next six months and we planted a couple of hundred trees and shrubs. We wanted to become self-sufficient, so most of what we planted were fruit and nut trees. It was all hard physical work but very enjoyable and it was the change we had been looking for. Our dream was becoming a reality. When the house was ready and after researching various options for a business, we chose to start a herb farm. We became members of a local, organic herb growers' network and were going to grow culinary herbs which would be transported to Sydney and Melbourne to be sold. I did some training with the network to learn about herb farming and prepared a large area of our land to be used for a herb garden. The fact that the street we lived on was called Basil Road, we took as a sign that this was the right choice.

In our eyes, Nimbin was also a very spiritual place. Almost everyone was into some kind of spiritual awakening through yoga, meditation and a myriad of religions and beliefs. We loved this environment and continued in our own development with new fervor. I meditated at least once every day and also started to see visions of catastrophes, usually in the form of great floods and sometimes knew what was going to happen before it actually did. That was pretty cool. Jenny and I talked non-stop about our spiritual experiences and everything we did and thought had a spiritual meaning. We listened to various Indian gurus that had followers in the area and became convinced that there were many ways to God and we all had to follow our own path. Jenny became more and more psychic and started to take a leadership role in the family. She was the one who often saw the future and knew what to do. She had very convincing arguments and I usually ended up agreeing with her.

Since we were vegetarian, cooking was not easy. I had to learn about preparing balanced meals to make sure our food intake contained sufficient protein, minerals and vitamins, especially since I did a lot of hard work in the house and garden. It was quite a learning experience. Strangely enough this had begun with Mitchel a few years earlier. When he started on solid food, he refused to eat anything that had meat in it. We tried to feed him baby food with meat or chicken in it, but he just wouldn't eat it. When we gave him lentils with vegetable puree, he would eat to his heart's content but any meat he refused. Initially we didn't understand how he could tell the difference. All the food was pureed. But eventually we came to the conclusion that he must be psychic too.

Mitchel was two-and-a-half years old when Jenny became pregnant again. We were looking forward to the birth because it would give

Mitchel a new focus in life. He had become increasingly difficult and we were at our wits end how to deal with his tantrums. One day he threw a tantrum in a shopping center in Lismore, a city about half an hour from Nimbin. We had just finished shopping and he wanted something we didn't want him to have. He threw himself on the floor and screamed. We first tried to calm him but nothing seemed to work. Eventually we walked away pretending to leave him behind. He couldn't care less and continued his screaming. We ended up standing on the first floor at the balustrade watching him. While he continued his tantrum, people gathered around him and probably wondered where the parents were. It became increasingly embarrassing to own up to him, but when he saw all strangers around him, he stopped and sat up. Jenny and I looked at each other and wondered what to do now. Eventually we were going to have to get him from down there. Inside I was cringing and felt totally helpless and out of my depth. I had no idea how to handle my son but knew that this was not good. We picked him up and fled the shopping center. I don't think we ever went back there.

Shanti was born and her name suited her to a tee. It means peace in Hindi and was given to us by a new age psychic we visited regularly. Shanti was the total opposite of Mitchel and utterly peaceful. Jenny and I sometimes even fought over who would rock her to sleep. When she lay on our chest in the rocking chair, she would fall asleep in no time and so would we. It was so relaxing.

Having a sibling did calm Mitchel down as he became involved in looking after her. Jenny was now completely absorbed with both kids and our relationship grew cold. There was very little physical contact between us and Jenny seemed to get irritated whenever I touched her. Sex was no longer on the agenda but abstinence was all part and parcel of eastern religions, so I accepted it. While she was focused on the children, she did less and less housework and often told me she had to relax. I didn't understand this - even after a twenty minute shopping trip to town, she needed to sit down and usually didn't get up for ages.

I didn't realize at the time that her mind was keeping her so busy that she didn't have any headspace to do anything.

Now when Mitchel was born I believed that he was in fact a gift from God and from the time that he could speak I believed everything that came from his lips was directly from God. Or I would find a way to interpret what he said as being highly significant and very spiritual. For example, when he pulled the dog's tail or tormented her, I would say

"Well the dog was put on this earth to entertain Mitchel"

or I would find a way to justify what he was doing spiritually. Nevertheless, he really did do some truly wonderful things as well. He was the one person who had great compassion for both me and others, but not for the dog. Whenever I was feeling unwell or depressed, he knew exactly what to say to make me or that person feel much better. No matter how young he was.

I began to look to alternative medicine. Homeopathic treatment was all around so I sought out the best. This man was a homeopath as well as a chiropractor and also had a practice in Brisbane. I was pregnant and he said that my hips were out of alignment and that some regular adjustment would result in a much easier birth. Much to his kind and generous nature most of the treatments were discounted or even free. I saw him once a fortnight for the entire pregnancy and true to his word the labor was only two hours and apart from a little back pain soothed with hot towels, my daughter's birth was as smooth as any birth could possibly be.

Shanti, as predicted by a guru we visited before she was born, was peaceful and content, the total opposite of how Mitchel's entrance to the world was. If she was tired and crying, I just said:

"It's OK, Shanti, you can go to sleep now"

and with a little rocking motion she would be asleep. A more blissful child you could never hope for.

There was a little Christian church in town and one day Jenny felt she was called to go and talk to the pastor in the hope we could unite our beliefs and work together. We wandered around the church and rang the bell of the pastor's house. He wasn't there so we left our phone number with his wife. He called us the next day and came for a visit. We weren't sure what we were going to tell him but we just wanted to connect. We talked for an hour about religions but he was not interested in any other religion than Christianity. We thought he was narrow-minded and I was annoyed that he was playing with a little cross on a chain that he held in his hand during the whole discussion. At the end, he asked if he could pray for us and we said that was ok. He prayed the blood of Jesus over us and the house, something I didn't really understand at the time. While he was praying this, I laughed inside. I was so convinced that I was right and he was wrong to believe in Jesus only. Afterwards, I was somewhat confused about the fact that he was such a nice man while I felt so angry with him. I was supposed to be at peace with all religions and have compassion for all but he irritated the hell out of me. No surprise to say that we never went to the church and we never saw the pastor again.

When I was working in the herb garden one day and some of the herbs were almost ready to be cut, I suddenly realized I had had enough. I was sick of talking to plants and my back ached again from bending over. What is it that is missing here? Why am I not satisfied with fulfilling this dream? And then it hit me like those few precious times in life when you get an insight into yourself that changes your whole perspective: I missed people. I am a people-person. I want to go back to teaching because then I'll always have people around. I want to work with people, not with plants. I decided in my heart that we were going to leave Nimbin and find another teaching job. A few weeks later, the final straw was when I went to town at seven in the morning to buy a newspaper. I parked the van and found an Aboriginal guy doing a rain dance on the pavement. He looked really out of it, most likely on drugs. I thought:

"This is not a good place to bring up children. It is time to go."

When I got back, I told Jenny my plans and she wholeheartedly agreed. She was always ready for a change. We decided to go to the Gold Coast. While planning our move, we became convinced we would 'find gold' there in the form of something incredibly precious. We sold the house and business in record time and left Nimbin.

CHAPTER 4 Back to teaching Canungra, Gold Coast Hinterland, 1992

Coming from the country it was very hard to settle in a city again so we decided to buy a house in a small country town in the Hinterland on the Gold Coast. The trees were close to the house and there were two mango trees in the garden which made us feel at home. The day we moved into the house was extremely hot. It was around forty degrees Celsius and the worst day to be moving. We rented a small truck and, with the help of a few of my new Japanese students, moved the furniture from a storage facility to the house. I was dripping with sweat all day long and utterly exhausted when we were finally finished in the evening. I sat down with a cold drink when a voice in my head said: "You won't stay here for more than nine months." I was used to these messages in my head but this one infuriated me. Why did we then have to move here on such a dreadful day to be moving out again in less than a year?

I had found a job teaching English as a second language at another Japanese owned college. The managing director was Japanese but the total opposite to Mr Honda. He was very quiet and laid-back and we hardly ever saw him. It was the principal, Ms Marjory Chung, who ran the college and supervised the teaching staff. How she got a Chinese surname I never found out. She was a typically British, grand-motherly type who gave a very friendly first impression and made you feel at ease. It was a small college with mainly Japanese students and I was surprised how easy it was to pick up where I left off a year and a half ago.

Jenny was not doing so well. I didn't work long days and was finished at one in the afternoon and was supposed to stay a bit longer to prepare lessons for the next day. However, she picked me up at one o'clock every day and needed me to take care of the kids and give her a break. I didn't really understand why, but when I asked her how her morning had been the standard answer was "Horrendous!" It started to both worry me and irritate me that everything seemed so difficult for her. I had seen plenty of other mums with young children now and they seemed to cope quite easily. Jenny had completely lost her sense of humour and everything was intensely serious. She was a different person from the woman I married ten years ago. She had lost a lot of weight again because she didn't eat much and she didn't look after herself. She often told me it had to do with this stuff that was going on in her head and we always linked it to her personal development and growth and thought that one day she would be perfected in her soul.

One night when we had just gone to bed, she grabbed me and said in a desperate voice: "Help me. I feel like there is nothing left in me. I have no personality like other people. Some women have lots of personality and they know who they are and they can talk and joke, but in me it's empty. There's nothing left and I can't live like this." She was crying and I said that I couldn't do anything about it. I was at a loss. Scenes like this freaked me out but I had to keep my calm and give her some kind of support. So I held her in my arms and hoped it would go away. It took a while but she finally settled down and fell asleep.

At other times, unusual things happened that showed me that Jenny was "in touch with the universe". One morning she woke up at five o'clock and told me we had to buy carpet today. The house needed to be carpeted but we hadn't shopped for it yet and hadn't even discussed the color. "I can see blue carpet and it's for us. Blue is the color of truth so we must get it. Today!" "Blue?" I couldn't imagine blue carpet in a house which was entirely in pine. All the walls and ceiling were pine and to have blue with all wood seemed to clash. Jenny was persistent and in the end I gave in and told her to shop around that day while I was at work. When she picked me up from work that afternoon, she showed me a sample of a beautiful blue carpet and when we held it against the wooden walls, it looked fantastic. It was a warm grey-blue and it was on sale with a substantial discount if we bought it that day. The sale was going to be finished the next day. We rang and ordered and when the guys came to the house to measure, they told us there was just enough carpet in store to cover all the rooms. I was amazed and had to admit that Jenny wasn't entirely off the planet. Some of the things she saw were quite real. After the carpet was laid, whenever someone came into the house, they would comment on the beautiful color and how well it suited the house.

Jenny spent most of the days on her own with the children and didn't make any friends anymore. She became more and more critical of other people and withdrew from all social contact. We hadn't had any family around for almost two years now and so we became very isolated.

Sometime earlier I remember that I had somehow come to the conclusion that if I was to be like Jesus I also had to go through life like he did. This also included dying like he did and suffering as he did on the cross. Only my suffering would be a mental degradation of my mind and then God would come and save me just in time. This I believed was his purpose for my life so that I would be able to come out of it all and help others through their confusion and suffering.

One night I was sleeping in bed and I could feel something tugging at my hands making me sit bolt upright in bed. Next I could feel this intense pain in my feet and hands as if I too had been nailed on the cross just like Jesus. It was not a dream, when I woke up completely, my hands and feet were extremely painful. I told myself that I had gone as far as I could go for God. This didn't ease the pain and suffering. I decided it was time to get some help. I found a local Homeopath since at that time we didn't trust doctors. She gave me a number of bottles of remedies and I believed this was to be my personal cure all. Initially I did feel better however not long after, I was back to where I started.

There were times when the stress of having to look after Jenny and two little children, work and doing most of the housework got to me. My days were busy but more than that they were stressful. As a result, I started having migraines. In the beginning they felt like a normal headache but there were times when I had to lock myself in the bedroom with the curtains closed while I was crawling around on the bed in agony. My head was pounding and I could feel massive tension in my neck. I knew it was a result of the stress of quite a few years now and so I found a masseuse who could massage my neck and shoulders and give me some relief.

Canungra was not what we expected. It was a boring little town and the people were not very friendly. We also ended up having to drive to the coast, about thirty minutes one way, for everything we needed and the driving was getting to us. We decided to move to the Gold Coast and live in the suburbs. We had lived in Canungra for exactly nine months.

CHAPTER 5 A horrendous day Nerang (1), Gold Coast, November 1992

The new house in Nerang was wonderful. It was in a quiet street. It had a brand-new kitchen and a huge living room at the back which looked out on a large backyard. It was ideal for the kids. I was also much closer to work and Jenny closer to the shops and other facilities. There was a medical center about two minutes up the road.

The changes seemed to have a good effect on Jenny's mood. She always loved changes and became alive when we moved to a new environment. She'd shop for all the bits and pieces we needed to make the new house livable and she'd move furniture around almost daily until she was satisfied that it was perfect. Although her behavior was a bit obsessive, it was a great relief that she was more cheerful. Unfortunately, this didn't last long and some days it was back to deep depression and "I had a horrendous day." Her moods began to swing. At times when she was really down, I would sit with her and talk to her to get her to focus on the good things in life.

"You have two beautiful children who love you and they are healthy and happy. This is because of you, because you are a good mother. You're doing a great job with them. I've got a job, I only work until 1.30 every day and we have enough money now."

Sometimes I spent an hour before she would finally pick up and smile again. However, it wouldn't last long. One evening after a long pep talk, we were laughing aloud for the first time in ages. It was a wonderful experience to have Jenny back the way she used to be. We used to laugh a lot together about silly little things and I always loved it that she enjoyed my sense of humour. After this good belly-laugh we got up and Jenny went to the bathroom. A few minutes later, I wondered what she was doing and I looked around the house. I found her sitting in a heap on the floor next to our bed. She was sobbing away and told me that she felt so rotten.

"But we were just laughing. I don't understand. What happened?!"

I was confused and Jenny's answer didn't really explain anything.

Life became increasingly difficult and stressful. I never knew what to expect when I came home from work. Occasionally parts of the house were cleaned up but over the next months it became more and more untidy. I desperately tried to keep on top of the housework but Jenny was so disorganized that it took me the whole weekend to bring some order into the place. I started to find dirty clothes and nappies and wet towels in the strangest places. It seemed that she dressed and undressed the kids and herself all over the house and then left clothes and nappies there. I found left-over food everywhere and even banana peels in between the cushions of the couch. Many things went missing. I couldn't find some of the kitchen utensils and some of the kids' toys. I assumed they were somewhere in the stuff on the floor in one of the rooms. Washing-up piled up on the sink and bags of rubbish sat on the kitchen benches for days.

Jenny became very uncommunicative and it was hard to get her attention. When I did and asked her to please wash up, we usually ended up in arguments. She told me she did housework all day long and was tired of it at night. I should do some and see what it was like. She became more and more critical of me. Nothing I did was good enough. One day, I asked her numerous times to wash up and she kept saying she would do it in a minute. She was sitting in the living room on the floor playing with the kids as usual. They were making some kind of cut-and-paste collage. I really needed her to help, because I had so many other things to do and I wanted to cook dinner. I noticed I just wasn't getting through to her and finally did the huge washing up myself. When I was finally finishing up, she came into the kitchen and looked at the sink. I was just emptying it when she criticized me about not wiping it.

"Look how dirty you leave it. You do this all the time. Can't you wipe it properly?"

I was flabbergasted. How dare she criticize me, while she does nothing all day? She was the most difficult person I had ever met in my life and I was married to her! I couldn't cope anymore; this is ridiculous! I told Jenny that if the kids were hungry, she could give them a sandwich and that I had to go for a walk to think. I was so angry – angry with her and angry with God. I walked to a nearby park and sat down at a picnic table. I looked up at the starry sky and screamed in a whisper:

"Oh God, help me! You've got to have something better for me than this!"

After I sat there for a while and had cooled off, I walked back home. I didn't expect anything to happen as a result of this desperate prayer.

On one occasion, I asked Jenny to get some shopping. For some reason, she was usually capable of doing this. I gave her a shopping list of about four items that I needed for dinner that night. She left and I stayed home with the kids. They were playing and watching TV so I could continue with cleaning and washing. Jenny didn't come back for about an hour and a half. I started to worry and kept praying. When she finally got home, she told me she had had a great time. She bought some clothes, a pot plant and another decorative trinket for the lounge room. It would look really nice.

"What about the food?"

She gave me a puzzled look and said:

"Food? Oh I forgot" and wandered casually out of the kitchen. On another occasion, I asked her to get some shopping before I went to work. When I got home at dinner time and asked her if she went shopping, she told me she had gone to the shops but hadn't been able to get anything. There was a woman in the supermarket with her little son who was pulling things off the shelves. After a few warnings, she had enough and she yelled at him:

"Don't do that!"

Jenny took this as a word from God and so she left the supermarket and went home. The words spun around in her head all day and she hadn't been able to do anything.

I had no idea what to do about all this. Jenny's reactions were often the opposite of normal. She could drink very strong coffee and then fall asleep. Most of the time she was not hungry but occasionally she ate a meal and told me:

"The more I eat, the more hungry I feel."

Often when I convinced her to eat, there was something wrong with the food. It had usually something to do with 'the energy' – the food had bad energy and made her feel sick. She could take one tiny bite of potato and this would make her feel ill and spoil her mood for the next five hours. In the meantime she bought masses of vitamins to help her with her health. She had also been breastfeeding Shanti for way too long and while Shanti was turning into a healthy looking, even chubby, toddler, Jenny was skin and bones. She started having unusual symptoms like a heavy weight was bearing on her chest or wet feelings on her legs and often went to the doctor.

What really freaked me out was that I noticed at night lying next to her that she often stopped breathing. I had to remind her to breathe and she would vaguely acknowledge and take a breath but it was usually irregular. Eventually one doctor put her on an anti-depressant and convinced her to stop breastfeeding. There was some improvement but it didn't last. When the doctor suggested she should see a psychiatrist, she never went back to him. There was no way she was going to see a psychiatrist, she wasn't crazy. She still believed that she was going through deep personal development.

She started to get up in the middle of the night. When I woke up and noticed she wasn't in bed, I got up. I found her pacing the living room and mumbling to herself or rolled up in a ball on the rocking chair crying and looking hopelessly lost. We talked for hours during those nights. She related to me how, when she was young, she was sexually abused a number of times by different guys – some were complete strangers and some friends of the family. It had started when she was around twelve years old, when she got into a car with a stranger who was going to give her a lift home. He molested her and she freaked out. She managed to escape and run home, but she never told anyone. Later she was sexually abused by a good friend of the family who would look after her and her sisters when mum and dad were out. This abuse went on for a long time and scarred her for life, she said. There were other minor incidents and she was going through them, re-experiencing them one at a time.

In New Age thinking, you regress, express the emotions around the traumas and then release them. This way you are supposed to be freed from deep-seated and repressed childhood traumas and subsequently move on with your life as a new person. I had experienced this myself many times so I knew how this process worked. It had released me from my own painful experiences from the past and I did indeed feel tremendously relieved. In fact, after I had remembered some of the things that had happened to me, hit some pillows in anger and cried through the memories, certain physical pain was released and never came back. I had suffered severe eye strain for many years and it had become increasingly unbearable. When I expressed the emotions, I discovered a painful childhood memory. However, when I worked through it, the issue was resolved. I no longer felt the eye strain and it never returned. I also felt immensely relieved inside and found a new joy.

The problem with Jenny was that there never was any long-term relief. She continued to go through the same traumas and didn't seem to be able to let them go. She was up for many nights in a row and after a couple of weeks of this I gave up and stayed in bed. There was nothing I could say that helped her and I needed the sleep. She actually agreed with me and said she would sort it out herself. However, one day I did finally convince her to see a psychiatrist. The problem was that psychiatric help was not covered under Medicare and extremely expensive. One of the doctors had recommended a psychiatrist who was also a General Practitioner so he was able to claim his consultations on the government and we wouldn't have to pay. We went there early one morning when Jenny was in a very agitated state and waited around in the car park under the building for the office to open. Jenny was pacing and wanted to leave. I persuaded her to wait; it was a quarter to eight and it would only take fifteen minutes. They finally opened the door and we had to wait because there was someone with an appointment at eight. We sat in the waiting room for about twenty minutes and I kept an eye on the door of the doctor's office. Eventually two men came out and I wondered if I could tell which one was the psychiatrist and which one the patient. One was dressed in badly matched casual clothes with messy hair and a beard and the other in a suit with no tie. His hair was in order and he was well-shaven. Looking at the expressions on their faces I guessed the guy in the suit was the doctor because he looked quite at peace and more together. When they got to the reception desk, they shook hands and the man in the suit left. Oops, I thought, I was wrong. However, I kept an open mind and we were called in. He was a nice enough guy but spent the whole time talking about my background instead of Jenny's. He said he would get to that later. However, we needed something immediately for her to calm her down. He said he couldn't just give her anything without finding out more and this would take weeks because he was very busy. He could see us once a week and slowly diagnose the situation. We left very disappointed and never went back.

I was seeing visions, many of which I have forgotten. I found that I could talk to the children's toys. Then all at once I heard an audible voice say that they were evil. I loaded up the car boot with everything and anything that was evil, as I saw it, including some of the children's much loved toys and Luke's favourite kitchen knives and tools. I took a drive and decided to take all the stuff to the dump. However, I got lost and couldn't find it so I ended up stopping on the freeway and throwing out everything in the bush.

Jesus appeared to me in a vision. He stood outside the house and looked at me sorrowfully. His image was like that of water quivering as he stood there, and I knew that the only way to be rid of this entire barrage of lies, pain and anguish of living with this intolerable manifestation would be to go and find Jesus. I knew beyond a shadow of a doubt that only He could give me the answers that I sought.

CHAPTER 6 Flavor of the month
Nerang (2), Gold Coast, 1993

When I drove to work in the morning, I said a prayer to protect my children and Jenny. I was starting to fear the things she did during the day. I had no idea and we had nobody to keep an eye on her. We had no friends and the closest family was hundreds of kilometers away. They didn't really know what was going on and I didn't know how to talk about what was happening. I was on my own. While driving, I often got that annoying little song in my head "Jesus loves me". Mitchel brought it home one day after Jenny had taken him to a Sunday school in Canungra. I didn't know why I had it in my head but it wouldn't leave me for weeks on end. I finally just started singing it although I didn't really agree with the words and would change them to fit my own ideas.

At work things were changing, too. Marjory turned out to be very moody and unpredictable. When a teacher did something that she didn't like, they would be severely reprimanded or even fired on the spot. This sent a ripple of fear and insecurity through the college and everyone was on edge. There was a rumor going around that I was in trouble with her too over something I had done and when I arrived at work one morning and ran into Marjory, she gave me a cold look when I said good-morning. I was very worried because I really couldn't afford to be out of work. As an ESL teacher I didn't make much money but it just covered our expenses, so losing my job would be disastrous. The next day I found a letter in a college envelope in my in-tray. I froze. This was the way people were called into Marjory's office and either told off or sacked. With my heart pounding in my throat, I opened the envelope and read the letter. I was asked to come and see Marjory and the managing director at the end of next week. Shit! I couldn't wait that long. I needed to know now. I talked to the secretary but she told me that Marjory had just gone overseas and would be back on Friday the next week. There was nothing I could do and I forced myself to put the issue out of my mind.

By the time next Friday came around, I had decided not to be intimidated by this woman. I was still very nervous, however, when I walked into her office. She smiled at me, said a very friendly hello and shook my hand. The Japanese managing director just sat there quietly. In a very pleasant voice she accused me of not fulfilling my contractual duties. She didn't give me any details and I decided it would be better not to ask. I had learnt with Mr Honda in the previous job that it was sometimes better to keep quiet when you talk to irrational people, especially when they are your boss. Marjory became uncomfortable because I didn't try to defend myself and after some awkward silence dismissed me. I smiled inside when I left her office and felt triumphant that I had manipulated her in a way that she constantly manipulated us and, anyway, I hadn't lost my job.

Two weeks later I found another letter in my in-tray. What now? I sat down in a quiet corner of the staffroom and opened the letter. What a surprise it was to read that the management wanted to offer me a promotion. The college had won a contract from the government to run English language courses for migrants to Australia and they wanted me to run the program. I was invited to an interview to discuss the details of the position. When I had time to think it over, I became very excited about the prospect. As a migrant myself, I had learnt Australian English and had adapted to the culture and it would be great to share that experience with others. The students would also be from many different countries and probably more mature than the young Asian students I was teaching now. On top of that, it meant a pay rise which would be very welcome.

In the interview I was told that despite my previous carelessness about my duties, management had decided that I was the right person for this job. Marjory's tone of voice was extremely patronizing and she made me feel that I should be utterly grateful that the college gave me this opportunity. This made me almost decide against accepting the offer, but I said I needed to think about the position and talk to my wife. It involved longer hours of course and a lot more responsibility. Marjory looked worried when I left the office. I think she was surprised I didn't say 'yes' straightaway. Again I smiled inside. I had already decided to take the job, but I enjoyed playing this game. I did actually have to talk to Jenny because she would have to be on her own for more hours every day. The job was nine to five.

To my surprise Jenny agreed immediately that I should take the job. I expected I would have to convince her and had all the arguments prepared. However, I didn't have to say anything. She thought I deserved this promotion and understood that it was perfect for me. It gave me hope again that she was actually recovering and getting back to normal. Because I was constantly dealing with irrational people, my life had become very insecure and I started to long for normality. This was brought home to me one day when I was in the staffroom at work and one of my colleagues was on the phone to his wife. He had a very relaxed conversation with her and a few laughs. Before he hung up the phone, he asked her to put some beer in the fridge for him so he could have a cold one when he got home. This simple request was unimaginable in my marriage. Jenny had often argued that alcohol was evil and I shouldn't need any. I hadn't had a drink in years. This simple conversation just made me aware of what is normal and how far from normal my life was.

Jenny said she would cook a meal for us tomorrow to celebrate my promotion. The next day I officially accepted the position and signed the contract. The migrants wouldn't start for another two months but I would start setting up the program in four weeks. My colleagues congratulated me and agreed that I was the best man for the job, mainly because none of them wanted to work so closely with management.

They jokingly added that I now would be Marjory's 'flavor of the month'.

When I went home that night I was looking forward to the meal Jenny had promised me. However, she had had a terrible day struggling with things and hadn't been able to get it together. I hid my disappointment but tried to remember that she had been so supportive the night before. She would cook the meal tomorrow. The meal never eventuated and although she really wanted to cook something special for me, she had completely lost the ability to organize it. She was still regularly getting up in the middle of the night and spending hours on, what she called, 'processing stuff'. The following week, I could hear her wailing and murmuring in the living room at night. I got up and tried to comfort her and help her through it. However, there was no end to 'the stuff' that had to be processed and it went on and on. We were up for three nights in a row. I took days off work because I was exhausted from being up all night and listening to all the intense problems. I realized I had to make a decision. Jenny was no longer functional and I couldn't let her go on like this. I was going to take her to the mental hospital.

I went to see the pastor's wife at the church where our son went to school. Within a short space of time and some discussion, I willingly gave my life to Christ. I finally saw what it was like to be a child of God. I was sparkling in His immense beauty, no longer was He sorrowful but joyous. I loved Him so much.

As yet it was still far from being over. I went home and the demons were flying all around the outside of the house - hordes of them. Yet Jesus would not allow them in.

Finally my mental state broke and Luke decided that it was time to take me to the hospital. Even as we sat in the hospital, I couldn't believe that he was leaving me there.

CHAPTER 7 Salvation
Nerang (3), Gold Coast, 1993

It was a Saturday morning and I had organized for the kids to stay at our neighbors'. Mitchel occasionally played with the little boy next door. I told Jenny that we needed to go somewhere together. We were going to see a doctor for her. I didn't give her any details. We drove to the Gold Coast Hospital and walked to the mental clinic. I hoped she wouldn't notice the signs 'psychiatry'. I knew she was going to protest if I told her that I was going to leave her in a mental hospital and was very concerned that she would cause a huge scene. I tried to keep light conversation and distract her whenever there was a sign. My stomach was in a knot. This was the hardest thing I had ever had to do but I knew it was the only option I had. We arrived and I asked to see a doctor. I was glad I didn't have to say psychiatrist because Jenny would have tweaked. All went according to plan. We talked to a doctor, I explained some of Jenny's symptoms and we decided she should stay for observation. She looked like a little lost puppy when I told her I had to leave her behind. She was terrified. I tried to calm her but in the end had to pull myself away while a nurse tried to distract her. I ran outside and wept. Driving home I pulled myself together because I had to look after the kids and make sure they were going to be ok without mum.

After I talked to the kids and explained that mummy had to be in hospital for a while, we had quite a nice weekend. Despite the fact that I felt that I had lost my wife, I knew she was in good hands because I had heard that the Gold Coast Hospital psychiatric ward had an excellent reputation. It was very clean, light and quite pleasant in there. It was also a great relief that I didn't have to worry about what she was doing. Jenny had a habit of disappearing and I never knew what she was up to. Now I could focus on the kids and clean up the house. Of course, I felt utterly lonely because I had no one to share this with. I also wondered when on earth I was going to be able to go back to work; I couldn't take too many days off. Mitchel had started kindergarten at a Christian school nearby so I had only Shanti to look after. Jenny rang a few times that weekend and we talked. She seemed to be coping alright but didn't want to accept that she needed to be there. I asked her to have patience and just talk to the psychiatrist to see if he could give her some medicine so she would feel better.

On Monday morning I dropped Mitchel off and ran into Michelle, one of the mothers I knew. She was a petite woman who had six children. I knew she was a Christian because she had made friends with Jenny and Jenny had invited her, her husband David and the children over for lunch at our house one day. It had been nice to have people over for a change but we had almost ended up in an argument over who the real God was. They believed in the God of the Bible only, which really clashed with our belief. However, when she saw me, she asked where Jenny was. I decided to tell her the truth. She told me simply that she would pray for us and if I needed something, to call her. I had to go to work but I still didn't know what to do with my daughter. One of the kindergarten teachers who had heard from Michelle what had happened, offered to keep Shanti for the day and look after her. She said she was welcome for the next few days until I had something else organized. Shanti was listening in and her face lit up.

"Can I stay, daddy, please, please?"

I was so relieved that she wanted to stay, because I had no other choice. I thanked the lady profusely but had to leave in a hurry because tears were welling up in my eyes.

That night I got a phone call that would change my life forever. It was Michelle's husband, David. His wife had told him what had happened with Jenny and he said he had been through the same thing with his wife. He knew what to do and he offered to come over to talk to me. I said:

"Thanks, I appreciate it but I really need some time on my own to think things through."

He understood and we hung up. The last thing I needed was a Bible-pushing Christian to tell me what to do; I couldn't stand the idea. But then, just when I hung up the phone a small voice whispered in my head:

"You prayed for help in the park last week, remember! Maybe this is part of the solution."

Something broke in me and ten minutes later, I rang David back:

"Please come and talk. I don't know what to do and I can feel this heavy darkness in the house. I am exhausted."

"I understand what you are saying. I will be there in twenty minutes."

I put the kids to bed and waited.

It wasn't long till I heard the doorbell and let David in. He was a short, stocky guy with brown hair and seemed both peaceful and determined. He had brought his Bible and my first thought was:

"Oh no, here we go."

but then decided not to resist whatever was going to happen. In any case, I had no more strength in me to fight. He sat down at the kitchen table and I made him a cup of tea.

"I was thinking about a scripture on the way over." he started. "It was Psalms 121. Let me read it to you: "I will lift up my eyes to the hills – where will my help come from? My help comes from the Lord, the maker of heaven and earth." See, God will help you, you don't have to worry."

He continued reading the rest of the psalm and it was nice to listen to. He asked about Jenny and he explained that his wife had had a mental breakdown a number of years ago and how they had become Christians. I didn't understand why I had to become a Christian since all religions lead to God, but I let him talk. After half an hour, there was a knock on the door. I was annoyed because I really didn't want to see anyone. I desperately needed to continue this conversation with David. I opened the front door and was utterly surprised to see Jenny standing there. She had decided to come home because she knew I was struggling. The hospital had been good for her to have some time to think but she didn't need to be there anymore. I was actually so happy to see her and thought this was good timing. She also needed to hear what David had to say. We talked for hours and finally David suggested we'd pray together. He said he had a prayer that had helped him enormously and asked if we would like to repeat it after him. We agreed. It was what Christians call 'the sinner's prayer' and I realized while praying that I was committing myself to being a Christian. I was vaguely aware that I had been manipulated into this without a proper explanation but since I had decided that whatever happened tonight, had to happen, my resistance to Christianity had disappeared. After the prayer, David said that we were now Christians and he would give us a Bible the next day. If we had any questions, we should call him. He'd be there for us at any time of the day or night. He asked if he could pray over the house and we agreed. We saw him raise his hands in every room and pray quietly. He also wiped his hands over the windows and prayed over the kids while they were asleep. He explained that that was the blood of Jesus and that would keep the devil out. He was so direct and to the point and it really impressed me that he had driven over to our house from the other side of town after a long day's work and had taken his time to talk to us. What's more, his own large family had to do without him for a long evening. He went home at about eleven o'clock.

Jenny said:

"I told you to believe in Jesus. He's the One."

We went to bed with a feeling that this was a new beginning. I woke up in the middle of the night and, as was my habit, I checked the clock. I had a digital clock and the time was '1:21'. I smiled and thought this confirmed everything tonight. It felt like God was showing me He was really in control.

The next morning I woke up and thought:

"Now I am a Christian. What on earth does that mean? What have we been through? What about all the other religions and New Age?"

I had a thousand questions running through my head and I was going to find answers.

Late that afternoon, the doorbell rang. There was an older couple at the door. They said they were from the church in Palm Beach and I realized that David had sent them. They carried a few containers and boxes and I was wondering what was in them. They asked if they could come in and they put everything in the kitchen. There was fried rice, noodles and two small boxes of other food items. They simply said that their church wanted to help people and that we should let them know if we needed more. I was so taken by surprise that I was speechless and could only mumble some vague "thank you" before they left. Again tears welled up in my eyes because I just wasn't used to getting any help or in fact anyone caring about our problems.

CHAPTER 8 The Gold Nerang (4), Gold Coast, 1994

When I went back to work, I was called into Marjory's office straightaway. I had phoned the college the week before to say that I needed time off work and had told the Director of Studies that I had had to take my wife to the psyche clinic. She was a very understanding woman and told me to take my time to sort out the problem. She asked if she could tell Mrs M, as she called her, and I agreed. I was beyond caring about Ms M's opinion. When I saw Marjory, she seemed in two minds about the situation. She started off in a friendly tone and asked how Jenny was. After a short explanation, she made this involuntary prophetic statement:

"So you have been to hell and back."

I hadn't told her about my giving my heart to Jesus, so she couldn't have understood the reality of her statement. However, she was concerned that I would not be able to take up the new position because I had to understand that this was a crucially important program for the college as it would bring in a lot of money. Government programs were well-paid, so she had to make sure I was up to the job. We were also competing with TAFE, the Australia-wide government institute of higher education that had just opened their beautiful new premises on the Gold Coast with state-of-the-art facilities. I assured her that things were now fine at home and I would definitely be one hundred percent focused on making the program a success. It didn't take too much to convince her because she had nobody else who was either interested or qualified to do this job. I knew I could do it and was really looking forward to it.

Ms M also noticed I hadn't shaved for a few days. Sometimes I just couldn't cope with these annoying routine tasks while my life was in such a mess, so I just let it grow. She wasn't sure what to say so I helped her out:

"I have decided to grow my beard, just for a change."

Her look of disgust almost made me burst out laughing but I was just able to suppress it and smiled.

"It'll look better when it is fuller."

Ms M was not convinced and responded:

"I don't like beards."

We left it at that. I knew that she couldn't ask me to shave and she knew it too. I let the beard grow for a while, and then trimmed it and kept it short. Reactions from colleagues were mixed; some said it looked distinguished, other said it looked scruffy. However, I started to realize that with the total lack of control I had over my life, this was something I could control. It was strange but I had a desperate need to be able to control something in my life and the beard was the only thing I could think of. It became a symbol of my new life.

It was close to Christmas and the students were organizing a market in the college to sell second-hand items and home-made international food. They set up tables in the classrooms on the second floor and displayed their goods. It looked very colorful. On one of the tables I found a CD with Christmas carols and bought it. When I was reading the back of the CD cover, tears welled up in my eyes. The family who sang the carols traveled around Australia to let people know that "Jesus really loves you." This touched me and I felt intensely happy with my new-found faith. Jenny and I realized that our salvation was 'the Gold' we knew we would find on the Gold Coast.

In the meantime, I read the Bible everyday. I needed answers. I thought I had followed God for the last ten years but now realized that it was not God. So who was it? Who was that Indian guru I had followed and seen in visions during meditation so many times and performed all kinds of miracles? What about Hinduism, Buddhism and the New Age? And what about the Roman Catholic Church I grew up in and ran away from? I had thousands of questions and just wanted to know the truth about God. I studied the Word, went to church and joined a home group. Scripture after scripture would answer my questions. "The devil can appear as an angel of light." hit me like a bombshell. This was my first revelation and I started rebuking the Indian guru. He was now attacking my house in the spirit and accusing me of betraying him. I told him that he had lied to me in the first place, that he was not God and that he was no longer welcome. I was now a child of God through Jesus Christ and no one else. I continued to put the blood of Jesus on the windows and eventually the attacks stopped.

In the first week after salvation, all the pictures of gurus and other religious figures were taken off the walls and we had a major clean-out. I went through hundreds of photos and all my writing and threw out everything that reminded me of the New Age and other religions. This included a box full of cassettes of New Age music and chanting and two boxes full of books. Jenny and I decided to burn some of the books and posters so we wouldn't be spreading all these lies and also as a symbolic gesture. In the process of doing this, we realized that we had to change our daughter's name. Shanti was a typical Indian name that reminded us of the Hindu religion and the New Age, so after some deliberation and consulting with the kids, we all decided on Chantelle. It means singer in French and it reflected her lovely personality. She was always singing songs she had learnt at kindergarten. We put in the paperwork to the birth and marriage registry and started calling her Chantelle. About six weeks later it was official.

Then I read in the Word that it didn't matter to God what we ate as long as we said grace and also that, after Noah came out of the ark, God told him that "every moving thing that lives shall be food for you." I told Jenny and we started eating meat for the first time in five years. It was liberating.

David checked in regularly by phone to see if we were ok. Some more discussions followed. My most urgent question to him was:

"You have five sons. How do you keep them under control?"

Mitchel had become quite unruly again. He had started at a Christian pre-school but came home with the foulest language. He wouldn't listen to any correction and was constantly pushing Jenny around. He also argued endlessly, and very intelligently, about everything we asked him to do. I wanted to know what the Bible said about this. I was shocked when David told me that he used a stick to discipline his children. The Bible calls it 'the rod of discipline'. He had learnt it from his father when he was young. He sat his children down and told them about the kind of behavior that was unacceptable in their family and that, if they behaved this way, they would be smacked. He showed them the scriptures in the Bible and told them that God expected this of him as a father, so that his kids would grow up as good kids. He did this because he loved them. This was my responsibility because I was the head of the household. You smack on the bum only and it must hurt, otherwise it won't work. Never do it in anger but only out of love. And finally, he told me that he didn't want to use his hands because his hands were used to reach out in love, to hug his kids and he didn't want them to be confused.

The next day I sat Mitchel down at the coffee table. I put a stick on the table and told him that there were going to be some new rules. I explained what was expected of him and everything else David had told me. Mitchel sat there listening intently and only said "Yes, dad" a few times. To my surprise he didn't argue. In the next couple of months I had to use the stick a few times. At first he resisted and after one smack threw himself on the floor and screamed excessively. I told him he had to stop or I would give him another smack. He didn't stop and I smacked him again. He needed to know I was serious about this. The discipline totally turned Mitchel's life around. He now had clear boundaries and he started to thrive within them. He became much calmer and would listen to instructions from both Jenny and me. It completely changed the atmosphere in our family. This was my first lesson in how powerful the scriptures are and that God's ways are often so different from our ways. Mitchel told me many years later, when he was seventeen, that he appreciated the fact that I had disciplined him. He was convinced that if I hadn't, he would have grown up a spoiled brat.

Jenny was doing much better. She seemed to be more at peace and was able to handle day-to-day affairs better. She had started counseling sessions at the church and was very impressed with the ladies that counseled her. She got all her questions answered and was learning just like I was. We had a lot to share and it was wonderful to be able to discuss these things with each other. I felt like my wife was returning to me after a long absence. After church we would have lunch together and talk about the sermon. She also started to look after herself again by combing her hair and putting on some make-up. There was still a long way to go, but things were looking up. One day after church, we went to the beach for a picnic. When we arrived at the beach, a powerful anointing came over me and I felt incredibly peaceful. This was so different from the peace I had felt during meditation. That kind of peace you had to work for. This new peace came from outside not from my own work. I almost floated onto the beach and I heard a gentle voice in the waves reverberating:

"I am that I am. I am that I am. I am that I am."

In the following months we continued going to church and joined a home group. Every sermon at church seemed to be relevant to my present situation and it was like God was speaking to me directly. When I walked into church the first time I noticed how the women seemed to be glowing. They looked so happy and healthy to me. Looking at Jenny, there was such a huge difference. I started praying for God to make her healthy and beautiful again.

Home group was run by two down-to-earth couples who were a little bit younger than us, but they became good role-models. They knew the scriptures really well and knew how to apply them to our daily lives. The guys also had a great sense of humour which lightened my heavy feeling. I looked forward to going every week because I was learning so much. Jenny also enjoyed the group.

A couple of months went by with relatively few problems and I started to trust that this Christian God was the real thing. I had started my new job and absolutely loved it. I was in control of both English language and literacy programs and had three teachers working for me. The migrants were a refreshing change because they were so much more interesting to talk to than the young Asian students. In the meantime, I had indeed been 'flavor of the month' and Mrs M was extremely helpful and positive. The meetings with her were conducted in a very friendly atmosphere and I could ask for whatever I needed to make this program a success.

Unfortunately, all this wasn't to last long; slowly but surely, Jenny's state of mind was deteriorating and she started to disconnect with reality again. She found it harder and harder to deal with everyday chores and the house became messier and messier. I had no control over this and our improved life was like sand slipping between my fingers. Jenny's facial expressions showed signs of severe stress; it was often twisted and she looked lost, bitter and overly critical. When we were in the swimming pool one day, I asked her if she wanted to jump into the water with us, but she said she couldn't and walked off. She was standing about twenty meters away and seemed totally absorbed in her own world. It was then for the first time that I thought she looked mentally ill. It shocked me that I recognized this twisted expression on her face but still didn't know what to do.

CHAPTER 9 Back to the hospital Nerang (5), Gold Coast, 1994

We kept going to home group but Jenny withdrew from the discussions and looked uninterested and pre-occupied. Her behavior became stranger again, too. One day on the way to home group in the car, she had taken two tops with her and couldn't decide which one to wear. She changed them about five times, while she was getting increasingly upset about the fact that she couldn't decide which one to wear. I couldn't convince her that both looked fine and that it didn't matter as long as she was comfortable. Her face contorted and I stressed out. She kept changing her top in the car. This was disturbing. At home group I spoke to one of the leaders in private and told him what happened and that things were not going well with Jenny. That night he had some intense prayer for her healing and peace. He laid hands on us and I could feel the anointing come over me. I always felt better after prayer.

In church I had been going up the front every time there was a prayer call and every time I would fall backwards and lay on the floor slain in the spirit for up to half an hour. I often wept and felt utterly lost and desperate inside. I was so exhausted from caring for Jenny and still didn't know what to do. Should I wait for super-natural healing or should I take her back to the mental hospital?

After we had been in the church for a few months, a baptism was organized for new Christians and we put our name down. We wanted to be baptized as a family as the next step in our Christian walk. We waited in anticipation and when the day finally came, we were very excited. When it was our turn, all four of us got into the little swimming pool that was set up inside the church building. There must have been at least two hundred people around the pool watching us. We went down under water together "in the name of the Father, the Son and the Holy Spirit" and I felt I dropped something in the bottom of the pool. I had my eyes closed and felt like I was floating when I became aware of a sudden stirring in the water and voices. I opened my eyes to see Jenny convulsing and making strange noises. I got on my feet to help her up. One of the pastors who had baptized us and was still in the water with us grabbed her and the other pastor who was outside the pool with a microphone started to rebuke a bad spirit in her. It didn't take long until she screamed and something came out of her. I saw a black, weird looking creature with flapping wings fly up to the ceiling of the church. It had an utterly confused expression on its face and seemed totally lost at what to do now. The pastor explained what had happened and we all praised God that Jenny was set free from this evil spirit. I was impressed that the pastors had immediately recognized the problem and had dealt with it so efficiently. We were in good hands. One of the home group leaders came up to me and despite the fact that I was soaking wet gave me a big hug. He said seeing us being baptized as a family was the most beautiful thing he had ever seen. It was a great blessing.

However, the situation wasn't to improve as yet. Although there was some kind of renewed feeling of freedom, Jenny was still not well. She had started some voluntary work at the kindergarten, where the children went, that was connected to the church and had been brought home early one day because she was feeling ill. When I got home from work, the doorbell rang and one of the kindergarten teachers was at the door. She told me they were very concerned about Jenny because they had found her in the little kitchen making really strange noises. She said they were all praying for her.

In the meantime, I had been getting regular phone calls from Jenny at work. She had this great need to talk to me and couldn't wait till I got home. It was usually about some great discovery she had made and sometimes about something that happened with the children. Since I was extremely busy at work, it became a burden to have to listen to her at times and when I heard my phone ring, I would worry that it was

Jenny with another weird discovery. Then one day it all came to a head just at the wrong time.

Normally I was in another building from Marjorie because there wasn't enough space in the original college. So my programs were run in another office block about a five minute walk away. I regularly visited the main college for meetings and to copy materials and borrow books. One afternoon, I was in the old building when the secretary told me that there was an urgent phone call for me. I was very concerned and asked where I could take a call in private. There were two phones in the staffroom but there were always a lot of teachers around. I was lucky that the manager was away that day and I could take the call in his office. I was petrified that Mrs M would see me go into his office and ask me what the problem was. I picked up the phone and was surprised that it wasn't Jenny. It was the lady from the kindergarten. She told me that Jenny had disappeared with Mitchel but had left Chantelle behind. She had phoned our home but Jenny wasn't answering even after half an hour. The drive from school to our house was only ten minutes. She was concerned that something had happened to Jenny and didn't know what to do. Neither did I. I didn't have a car and there was no way I could leave work two hours early and not alarm Mrs M. We decided she would phone home every twenty minutes or so and I would ring her to check. There was nothing else I could do. I prayed:

"OK, Lord, you got me now. There is nothing else I can do but trust in You and trust that You will look after Jenny and the kids. You got me cornered."

I started laughing aloud; it kind of bubbled up from the inside. I tried to continue work and pretend there was nothing wrong. Every half hour, I snuck into the manager's office and rang the kindergarten, praying that Mrs M wouldn't see me. Three phone calls later I finally heard the good news that Jenny had arrived home with Mitchel. The kindergarten teacher would take Chantelle home and come and pick me up at five o'clock. She had organized another lady to stay with Jenny until I got home. I couldn't thank her enough. I stayed at work till five and went outside. It was a dark afternoon and it was pouring down rain. It took half an hour for the lady to arrive; she had got lost on the way. My patience was being tested but I also felt that something had broken inside of me and my trust in God had grown. He had organized two wonderful women to take care of my family and this in itself was something completely new. I was still unused to getting help from anyone and had always been totally isolated with all our difficulties. Now God had put some people around me to help.

When we got home, Jenny was in the bedroom in a daze. She hardly recognized me and I decided that I had to take her back to the hospital. The ladies offered to help me in the next couple of days. The following day was Friday and I couldn't take time off work, so they would take the kids to school and stay with Jenny during the day. I would then take Jenny back to the hospital on Saturday while they would look after the kids until I picked them up. I had never been so grateful in my life and had tears in my eyes when they left.

The next two days everything went according to plan. It was hard to focus at work; I was planning how to take Jenny to the hospital without her realizing it. I knew she would resist tremendously because she hated the place. On Saturday morning we had breakfast together in the kitchen. Jen was aloof. In the middle of breakfast she got up and disappeared to the bedroom. The kids asked, as they often had recently, what was wrong with mummy. I said that I would tell them later and that they would be going to their friends' house today. Jenny came back with some clothes in her hands that she had recently bought. Without noticing us, she walked outside through the front door and I could see her throw the clothes into the big green rubbish bin. She came back in and got more clothes and toys from the bedrooms and walked them outside. I got up and followed her out and asked what she was doing. She said this stuff had to go.

"But it is all brand-new."

That didn't matter, it was no good. I gently took the items from her and put them back inside. I asked her to finish breakfast and emptied the clothes out of the bin. This confirmed to me that she had really lost it.

I dropped the kids off and took Jenny to the hospital. When we arrived she faintly protested but I gently encouraged her to trust me. We spoke to a psychiatrist-in-training and he asked her a few questions. He was obviously inexperienced and Jenny was so detached that she had no idea what the questions meant. She just agreed with everything he said even when he asked if she had thoughts of suicide. It was an awful interview but I was determined to leave her there until a proper diagnosis was reached. I told the trainee that I did not want her to leave until I gave permission. We were taken upstairs to the lock-up psyche ward and shown into a room. Jenny sat down and got very worried and started crying:

"You are not going to leave me here, are you?"

I held her in my arms and tried to comfort her.

"This is the best thing for you, darling. You have to be brave and stay here until we know what is wrong with you. You will feel much better soon. Just tell the doctor what is going on with you when you see him. Tell him how you're feeling and what is going on in your mind."

It was hard to calm her and eventually the nurse suggested I should just go. She was in good hands. I tore myself away and walked out of the ward and out the door that had to be unlocked for me to let me out. When I looked back my heart broke. I kept my emotions under control and started driving home. I was praying intensely for the Lord to look after Jenny and asking why this had to happen again:

"Lord, I thought you would heal her and now she is in hospital again, worse off than before."

I felt like I had really lost her this time. There was a car in front of me and for no apparent reason I looked at the number plate. It said 'CRY'. I couldn't keep the tears back any longer and wept uncontrollably. I continued to pray for a while until I heard the Lord's voice in my head:

"Look what I am going to do!"

I slowly calmed down as I realized that God was going to do something good. He was going to heal Jenny and make her beautiful and whole again.

When I picked up the kids, I was offered some lunch but I couldn't eat; I was stressed out. The ladies from the kindergarten promised they would look after the kids before and after school and I could pick them up when I came home from work. I thanked them and just couldn't believe the help I was getting. I took the kids home and sat them down on the couch with me. They wanted to know where mummy was, of course.

"Mummy is in the hospital and will have to stay there for a while until she gets better. "What's wrong with her?"

I tried to explain that there was a problem with her mind and her thinking and suggested we would pray together for God to make her better. I felt a surge of faith welling up in me and we prayed aloud holding each other close. Mitchel went quiet but Chantelle had to add her prayer as determined as a three-year-old could be:

"Yes, Lord, get rid of mummy's mind. Get rid of it in Jesus' name, Lord!"

Mitch smiled and so did I, but we knew God was listening.

The next days I visited Jenny in the hospital. We would meet in the common room and the first day the conversation was awkward. Looking at the other patients there, I was shocked to have to recognize how well Jenny fitted in. She looked so lost and disconnected from reality. After a few days she opened up a little. She seemed to be feeling more at home and was getting used to the routine in the ward. She also had a lot of time to think and talk to other patients. They talked a lot about Jesus and at least one in two had a Bible with them. She told me that she had seen Jesus:

"Really, He came and visited me. He was standing in my room and told me that everything would be OK."

She continued and was very intense about it. I wasn't sure how to take it. Could I believe this or was it a hallucination? She asked about the kids and I promised I would bring them the next day after work. She wanted to come home because she missed us so much.

On Sunday I went to church. Some key people seemed to know Jenny was in hospital again. They encouraged me, prayed for me and the counselors ensured me that it was the best thing for Jenny. She needed a good diagnosis and the right medication. They also told me that they would come to our house the next day and clean up while I was at work. I felt embarrassed about that and said that it wasn't really necessary. However, I couldn't convince them. They had already organized seven women to come and clean and prepare some food. This was one thing that impressed me no end with Christians: they were so practical and serious about helping us. We organized I would leave a key for them to get in.

On Monday afternoon I left work at five as usual, picked up the kids from the kindergarten-lady's house and took them straight to the hospital. There were a lot of hugs and tears but it was good to be together with the four of us for an hour. Then I told Jenny I had to take the kids home to feed them and put them to bed. She wanted to come home too but I convinced her to stay. She had seen the psychiatrist that day and he was a nice man. He had given her some pills to sleep at night. I promised I would come and visit everyday with the kids.

When we got home, I couldn't believe my eyes. The house was spotless. Everything was cleaned and organized, even the kitchen cupboards. There was a freshness in the house I had never experienced before. I rang the counselor to thank her and she told me they had prayed and worshipped in the house the whole day while cleaning. It was like a brand-new house. I was so thankful. When I hung up the phone, I opened the fridge to fix some dinner for the kids. It had been cleaned out and was stocked with food. Then the doorbell rang and there was one of the ladies from the church with a freshly baked pizza. I was overwhelmed and kept thanking her over and over. She handed me the pizza, told me to ask if I needed any help and left. It was the first time in days I ate something. It tasted fantastic.

The next couple of weeks were hectic: get the kids ready, drop them off, go to work, pick the kids up, go to the hospital, go home, prepare dinner, clean up and other housework, put the kids to bed. I would finally sit down and have some prayer before falling into bed exhausted. On the weekends we picked Jenny up and took her out to a park or even home. She looked out of place when we took her out and she actually asked to go back after an hour and a half. It was hard for all of us to drop her off at the hospital every time. One day, I decided to break the gloom and suggested we sing praise and worship songs while driving her back. We had all learnt a number of songs at church and started singing together. The gloom lifted immediately and we sang to our hearts' content. We could now say goodbye with a smile on our face. The Holy Spirit was definitely our comforter.

Jenny had seen the psychiatrist a few times now and he wanted to see me. I was very glad about that because I knew most about the situation and I couldn't be sure about what Jenny was telling him. I sat down and wrote a list of problems and symptoms I had noticed with Jenny over the years. I ended up with two lists – one with behavioral issues and one related to her thinking. The lists were quite long and I felt like an idiot that I hadn't taken her to hospital years earlier. When I met the psychiatrist, I was impressed that he was such a gentle person and a good listener. I explained my lists in detail. He complimented me on my analysis and told me that my lists confirmed his diagnosis.

"There are two kinds of mental illness" he explained. "One group of illnesses is related to our moods and the other group is related to our thoughts. The mood-related illnesses include depression and the thought-related illnesses include schizophrenia and other psychotic disorders. There is an overlap in the symptoms of these two groups of illnesses but they usually require different medication. In other words, the diagnosis is of crucial importance because if someone is diagnosed in the wrong group, he or she may be on medication for months or even years and feel no improvement. I understand that Jenny has been on anti-depressants for years?"

"Yes, that's right." I answered. He continued:

"Now your lists confirm my analysis. I think Jenny actually suffers from both illnesses. She has severe depression as well as schizophrenia."

The word hit me like a bomb:

"Schizophrenia?"

That sounded so serious. He noticed the stunned expression on my face and gently said:

"I don't know how you stayed with her for six years. Most men would have left because they are impossible to live with."

I left the hospital with mixed feelings. On the one hand, I was shocked to hear that Jenny was so seriously ill; on the other hand, I was greatly relieved that I finally knew what we were dealing with and could get proper treatment. The doctor had assured me that the latest medicines were excellent and that Jenny would be able to fully function when the medication had kicked in. I had to be patient for a few months but she would be fine. Also I could read up on it now and understand it better. The doctor had given me some brochures.

When I got home, one of the ladies from church was waiting for me with a few shopping bags. She was a large woman with a heart of gold. She had noticed that, when they were cleaning the house that the children didn't have a lot of clothes and had decided to buy some new things for them. So, we had a fashion show. The kids tried on the clothes: there were t-shirts and shorts for Mitchel and tops, a skirt and a lovely yellow dress for Chantelle. Again, I had tears in my eyes. I couldn't believe these Christians; they were so generous, not just with their time but also with their money. Chantelle was twirling around in her new yellow dress, smiling from ear to ear.

"Daddy, look at me!"

Mitchel was also very impressed.

"Look, dad. This t-shirt is cool!"

CHAPTER 10 Something not quite right

Nerang (6), Gold Coast, 1994

Reading the hospital brochure on schizophrenia, it struck me that Jenny had shown all the symptoms that were listed. She seemed to be a classic case of the illness. Apart from disconnecting with reality, withdrawal from social contact, hallucinations and voices, there was the unusual description "there is something not quite right". At first, it sounded strange to me but when I considered it for a while it was what I had often thought:

"There is something wrong, but I don't know what."

I had often noticed that this was how people reacted when they met Jenny. They looked at her like there was something not quite right. This was because her behavior and facial expressions were somewhat odd.

The brochure also emphasized the point that schizophrenia is definitely an illness that needs to be treated. Some people think that schizophrenics live in an alternative world and are just different from the rest of us. The brochure denied that they were just more sensitive and we should therefore accommodate them. Reading this I was aware that we had often thought this because we thought that Jenny was going through intense personal growth and we had to accommodate that. It was a relief to read this as I whole-heartedly agreed, and it even crossed my mind that I could have written this brochure myself.

After three weeks I was deemed to be OK and was sent home. They put me on a drug which caused my emotions to shut down. No longer could I feel the love of my husband or children. I felt locked up inside now. In my desperation I would stretch my arms out to feel the children yet nothing would come.

After three weeks in hospital, Jenny had stabilized on an anti-psychotic drug and an anti-depressant. Although she was still very vulnerable, she looked like a new person, could smile again and was at peace inside herself. She was ready to come home. I was advised to keep stress levels down and maintain calm at home. Stress could bring on another episode. Jenny needed a lot of rest and a feeling of security. She needed to be loved while she continued to heal. This should not be a problem, I thought. The previous week in church I had heard a sermon on marriage. While a woman should submit to her husband, the husband was to love his wife unconditionally like Jesus had loved the church and had even died for it. I realized that submitting to a husband was probably the hardest thing for a woman to do while the hardest thing for a man was to show this love to his wife. On the other hand, I became aware that since I hadn't really had a wife for years, I had a need to love her. My heart had grown cold towards Jenny and the idea of loving her again like I did in the first years of our marriage filled me with warmth.

It felt like starting all over again. Jenny had been through a total mental breakdown and was now slowly but surely turning back to normal. The experience of the last six years had changed both of us and we needed time to get to know each other again. Jenny was quite insecure about us. Although the memories of the last six years were blurred with big black holes, she recalled some of the things that had happened to her and started to wonder why on earth I was still with her. For me the memory lapses were a blessing but Jenny kept asking what had happened. She needed to understand. When I came home from work, she often told me what she remembered, then apologized to me about her behavior and asked me to forgive her. I told her over and over that I had forgiven her and that I was just very happy she had "come back". She continued the process of recovering memories and expressing her regret. One Saturday morning she told me that she remembered she had dropped a few bags full of toys and tools somewhere in the bush. She told me she had gathered all this stuff in bags because she thought they were evil and had dropped them somewhere along the freeway. She said she could probably find the place. We got into the van and drove there. I had a feeling that I should not have taken the kids but I didn't listen to that small inner voice and they came with us. I wasn't sure what to expect. Jenny told me to stop somewhere along the freeway and we walked into the bush. After about twenty meters we saw a number of plastic bags. When we opened them they were full of the kids' favourite toys, teddy bears, my tools and other possessions. Most of it was soaked and the kids looked at it in shock. I had to do some fast talking to put them at ease and told them they had to forgive mum because she was very ill when she did this. I promised this would never happen again. Jenny also apologized over and over but I blamed myself for being so stupid to take the kids with us. We cleaned everything up as well as we could and the kids were happy to have retrieved some of their old toys.

Despite some intense inner struggles and trying to control her thoughts, Jenny was improving slowly and was becoming more and more functional. She saw the psychiatrist on a regular basis and also continued with counseling at the church. After one of these counseling sessions she told me that they had discovered she was possessed with the ungodly spirit of this Indian guru we had been following for years. With intense prayer, they had started to deliver her but they aborted the process after two hours. There was something in the way of her being set free from this nasty spirit and they asked if I could come with her the next day. One of the counselors, who was very experienced in these things, had said that I had to be set free first since I was the head of the household. That night Jenny was very agitated and couldn't sleep. It was disturbing to see her that way again and I felt an intense anger welling up in me against this guru and all his false religion. I took the next day off work and went to church with Jenny. They prayed over me first to sever any relationship I might still have with this guru and had me confess that Jesus is Lord over my life. They then rebuked the evil spirit in Jenny and told him to leave. Jenny was slouched in an armchair and I could see the features of this guru reflected in her face and that he was holding on to her with his claws hooked in. I was sitting on the floor in front of the chair holding her feet and was praying intensely for release. This went on for twenty minutes but nothing seemed to change. When I looked up at Jenny, I saw that she was very passive and the words came out of my mouth:

"Jen, you have to take a stand. YOU need to tell him to leave you alone. Stand up for yourself! You don't have to take this anymore."

Jenny sat up straight and started to rebuke the guru's spirit and within seconds there was a visible change in her countenance. The evil spirit had left her and her face lit up. She was free. We thanked God for that and asked Him to fill her with the Holy Spirit. When we left the church, Jenny could hardly walk. She was drunk in the Holy Ghost and had to lean on me heavily. She looked like a new woman and was smiling all the way home.

Once I was delivered I felt utterly empty yet complete in myself. As I was sitting on the floor I became suddenly aware of what I had just gone through, an incredible experience and as time passed it occurred to me that what I had been through was actually very scary indeed. Prior to my deliverance I wasn't aware of there being anything wrong with me. Yet now that I was set free I could know myself entirely. It still took quite some time to adjust to the new awareness of myself. After all, after such a powerful deliverance and realizing what had just happened I became intensely afraid of the spirit world and how I had been misused by it. I decided that I didn't want any more spiritual experiences and that discerning good from evil was not that easy. I didn't want to be misused again. However, much later, discerning the spirit of God and His anointing was not something I wanted to miss.

After the deliverance, she started to look after herself once more and looked quite pretty again. She ate regularly and put on some weight. I was over the moon. Life had finally become normal. We could go out and do things as a family. Just taking the kids to a playground was a delightful experience. It was normal. There had been so many times that I had craved normality – just a normal meal together, a normal shopping trip and a normal reaction from a normal wife. It was wonderful to hear Jenny say that she was so happy to see me when I came home from work. I had a wife again and a wife I could love and who responded to that love. One day when we were in the kitchen and Jenny was struggling with her thoughts and insecurity around our relationship, I told her that I would stay with her and I would never leave. I asked her to trust me. I said I had stayed with her through all these years and it could not possibly get more difficult than it had been. We recommitted ourselves to each other, almost like redoing our wedding vows and I could feel a strong anointing come over us when we hugged. This was God's approval of our commitment. We both laughed with tears in our eyes and felt this was a very important moment.

When you are in the middle of a healing process, it often seems slow-moving. Can't the Lord hurry up a bit? Can't He heal her instantly? I knew He was all-powerful and that He could do whatever He liked. At times it was all a bit slow for me. On the whole Jenny was recovering but sometimes still suffered from strange symptoms. Her vision was blurring and there was occasional dizziness. There was still something not quite right. The psychiatrist had a suspicion and wanted Jenny to have a CAT scan. This sounded alarming but Jenny didn't hesitate to go to the hospital and have it done. Again we had to wait. The result would be available in a week. It seemed to me that some weeks were longer than others. I kept myself busy at work and tried not to think about it. Finally the day came and Jenny went back to the doctor to get the results. When I got home, I was told the news that she had a one-inch long brain tumor but they didn't know yet whether it was malignant or not. Jenny didn't seem too upset. She was convinced that the Lord was going to look after her. I succeeded in keeping calm on the outside but on the inside I was in turmoil. Hadn't we been through enough already? Why did God allow this to happen? And why just now when things were finally getting better? Why me? Why us? Why so life-threatening? The questions were racing through my mind and I felt I had no answers. That night when Jenny had gone to bed, I grabbed my Bible and stood in the living room. The tears were running down my face while I prayed:

"Lord, I don't understand why this is happening but I hold up Your Word to You. Your Word tells me that Jesus heals us and took all our illnesses to the cross. I trust that You will heal Jenny of this tumor. I believe in Your Word rather than the word of the doctors."

Then the waiting began. The doctors had decided that they needed to have an MRI to have a better look at the tumor. An appointment was made in a hospital in Brisbane, one hour north of the Gold Coast because the Gold Coast hospital didn't have an MRI machine yet. The Brisbane hospital couldn't fit us in until two weeks later, so we had to be patient. On the weekend we went to church and the counselors had asked us if we wanted prayer up the front. There was power in communal prayer, they said. We agreed and went in front of the church. Some people joined the pastor, laid hands on Jenny and prayed for healing. It was a great feeling to have all these people gathering around us and supporting us. There was a strong presence of the Lord. Afterwards, one lady told Jenny that she could see the tumor shrink and disappear. Jenny took this as the truth but I was more skeptical. I needed to see the MRI result. The following two weeks crawled by slowly and the day finally came that Jenny had to go to Brisbane. After the MRI we had to wait again of course for the result. After a week we were going to see the doctor who had referred us to the hospital. When we entered his surgery, he was sitting there with the results in his hands. He looked at us and said:

"I don't know what happened but the tumor has completely disappeared."

What a relief! Thank you, Lord! We both smiled knowingly and I said:

"We know what happened. It's a miracle! We prayed for this."

The doctor was somewhat taken aback and mumbled:

"Well yeah, that could be."

When we told the psychiatrist the next day what had happened, he actually stated:

"This is a miracle! I believe that that sometimes happens."

When we went back to church that Sunday, we gave our testimony to the whole church and we all praised the Lord for His goodness.

The following week, I was watching a TV interview with a celebrity who had had a nervous breakdown. He was telling the interviewer that after three years of the breakdown, it was still extremely difficult to even get out of bed in the morning. He was on all kinds of medication and to do this interview was a major stressor for him. Everything in his life was still a struggle and it would take him years to get back to work if ever. I could see his hands were shaking and his facial expressions showed anxiety and anguish. I felt for him but also became acutely aware of how incredibly well Jenny was doing. She had had a much worse diagnosis than just a nervous breakdown but was coping so much better than this guy. If anything, the Lord was showing me here how His healing power works – maybe not instantly but definitely faster than in the world. When I told Jenny the next day, she just smiled and said:

"I know. I told you He was always with me even in the psyche ward when I was completely out of it."

When Christmas was approaching, the children were asked to participate in the yearly play at church. Every Saturday afternoon, they had to be dropped off at the church building for practice. Chantelle especially was thrilled to be involved as she loved singing and dancing.

For Mitchel it was more of a social occasion. He loved spending time with his new friends from church. Jenny and I would then go to the beach to 'walk and talk'. We had a lot of history and issues to work through and a new relationship to build. It was always better to be walking. After a long stroll, we would have lunch somewhere along the beach. We both looked forward to these few hours together since it was the first time in seven years we had some time without the children.

CHAPTER 11 Mrs M
Nerang (7), Gold Coast, 1995-97

While at home things were constantly improving, at work things were quite challenging. New groups of students had arrived at the college, most of who were from ex-Yugoslavia. I had Serbs and Croats in the same class. They sat at opposite sides of the classroom. This made me very nervous and it took me many weeks before I finally dared ask them if they were OK with it. To my surprise, one of them said that there was no problem.

"We left the war in our country and want to live here in peace. We saw so much trouble, but the old people who live in Australia for long time, they want fighting. We don't want."

All the others nodded in agreement. What a relief! However, I started to realize that quite a few of these people were deeply scarred by their war experiences. One morning, a fifty-year-old Croatian lady came to class late and looked very depressed. She sat down and within a few minutes broke down in tears. I had to stop my lesson and asked her if she wanted to share what was going on. The rest of the class was silent and looked at her. In broken English, she said she hadn't been able to sleep because of nightmares. She had lost her two children in the war. They had just disappeared one day. Then her husband and she went through a freezing winter with insufficient warm clothes and blankets and no heating. At some stage they were cutting their own furniture and trees in the street to burn. When they survived the winter, they were able to move to a camp in Switzerland and by some miracle, were reunited with her children. They had been caught up in some riots and somehow escaped to Spain where they had lived with a relative for two years. Other students added their stories.

Another time, a tough military officer from the Serb army blurted out in the middle of grammar lesson:

"In war, all my friends killed. I see them die."

This came out of nowhere and I asked him if he wanted to share his story. He did. Many migrant women also started sharing their stories with me. I just listened. It became clear that mental illness was rampant especially among the men who had been fighting in the war, had been captured and tortured. Some of the husbands were obviously suffering from depression and some of schizophrenia. I did some research and found Serb and Croatian psychiatrists who specialized in war trauma and, with Mrs M's permission, organized for the migrants to visit them. Unfortunately, the men who needed that kind of help most refused to go.

Mrs M was quite against me getting involved with our migrants' private lives. However, I convinced her that teaching had become quite impossible with all these personal difficulties in the classroom. I had just done my testing of their English language ability in the middle of the course. The tests were one-on-one and I had had five woman break down and cry. It was impossible to test them and instead I let them tell me their stories. One told me about her husband who was missing in Yugoslavia. She hadn't heard from him for two years. Another told me about her husband who was dysfunctional and extremely lazy. He couldn't sleep at night because of recurring nightmares about his torture. Another lady from Egypt told me about her persecution in Cairo because she was a Christian. She and her husband had lost everything and had fled the country. She wasn't coping in Australia. I ended up praying with most of these women because that was all I knew I could do. Later I heard that the Egyptian lady was in the Gold Coast hospital mental clinic and that the other lady was reunited with her husband who had escaped Yugoslavia unharmed. I felt that the Lord had put me in this job to listen to these broken people.

Mrs M withdrew and I didn't hear from her for at least six months. I was happy about that. The programs were running very well and the feedback from the students and the government department who sent them was very positive. Then out of the blue, I got a phone call from Mrs M:

"Why are you not following the program?"

"I am following the program. What's the matter? Is there a problem?"

I was surprised to hear her on the phone after so long and the question didn't make any sense. She accused me of not implementing the programs properly but gave me no detail or no indication where she had this information from. Finally she hung up the phone without any apology. Then one day I had to meet with her to discuss the dates of the next literacy course. The meeting itself was pleasant enough but I could sense a constant suspicion. We decided to start the new course in a fortnight and I was given the go-ahead to organize the details and inform all the relevant parties. I wrote a flyer and sent a copy to Mrs M. The following day, I decided to take my class to a coffee shop for the last lesson. This was a usual thing to do to promote conversation among the students in a different environment. It was a lovely day and we sat outside on the terrace. It was very enjoyable. After twenty minutes the waitress came over and asked my name. She said there was a call for me from a very angry woman. I had no idea who that would be. The phone was in the kitchen and all the staff's eyes were on me when I picked up the receiver. When I said hello, I heard Mrs M yelling:

"How dare you decide to start the literacy course in two weeks? Who told you to make decisions like that? And I have to learn this from a flyer?"

She was raving mad and all the kitchen staff could hear the screaming, because I had to hold the phone away from my ear. I felt extremely embarrassed and tried to calm Mrs M down. I told her in a soft voice that we had decided on that date together yesterday in the meeting. She obviously didn't remember this at all but didn't say so. She raved on for a while and then suddenly hung up. I felt bewildered but realized she was really losing it. There were rumors going around that she was using a cheap diet pill that she had bought in Thailand, which was similar to speed. She was hooked on this drug and it was obviously affecting her mind.

The college staff were very concerned about Mrs M's behavior and decisions. The college was in financial trouble but the Japanese managing director, Mr Takahashi, now named Mr T, did nothing. It seemed like he was just waiting to return to Japan to retire and was completely under Mrs M's thumb. Mrs M continued to bring in new people who were put on a pedestal for a short while and subsequently criticized for incompetence and eventually sacked. The new 'flavor of the month' was a young marketing manager who had no experience in education and seemed totally oblivious of cultural issues. He had never been to any Asian country and yet we were told that he was going to turn the college around by bringing in hordes of new students from Japan, Korea and Brazil. He spent long hours in Mrs M's office and looked exasperated when he came out. Mrs M was all over him and even wined and dined him like he was her latest hot new boyfriend. Being double his age, it was a sad sight and we felt sorry for him. She actually introduced him to all staff and embarrassed him greatly by stating how good-looking he was. She also joked about the fact that when she saw the yearly financial statement of the company that she thought the little red number down the bottom was profit, but found out later it was a loss. After long deliberations the director of studies, Geraldine, and I decided to write a letter on behalf of all staff to the management in Osaka expressing our concerns. We worded it carefully and we knew we were taking a great risk because Japanese companies have a very strong hierarchy and never speak to employees directly. All communication goes through all the layers of management before it reaches the employees. However, since our management was so incompetent we felt we had no other choice.

The new marketing manager made one trip to Asia and subsequently disappeared. We weren't even told what happened to him but we could guess. In the meantime, Mrs M had conjured up another brilliant marketing plan. She was going to find new students in Uzbekistan and Nigeria. She would be traveling with Mr T and would also visit Japan, Korea and Brazil. The flights alone cost $20,000 but this would be a great investment for the future of the college. Nobody had ever thought of marketing our courses in Uzbekistan and Nigeria and later they could include neighboring countries as well. Our mouths fell open. It was so obvious to us that nobody had ever marketed English language courses in these countries because people there had no money to come and study in Australia. In the meantime, a reply had arrived from Osaka but not to us. It was directed to the management. Geraldine and I were called into Mrs M's office and accused of going behind her back. She was extremely disappointed and would sack us if she wasn't about to take off on her long marketing trip. She couldn't afford to lose us right now so we should be very grateful. Mr T just sat there with a dumb smile on his face and said nothing. After the meeting, Geraldine asked me if she could come and teach in my department. She didn't want to be in charge of the whole English department when it would all collapse. She couldn't work directly for Mrs M any longer. I agreed and to our surprise so did Mrs M. So Geraldine moved to our building, away from Mrs M and taught the migrants. She felt greatly relieved.

When Mrs M and Mr T came back, they brought a couple with them from Uzbekistan. I was told they would be visiting my building and I should spend some time with them and show them around. They were owners of a small English language college and Mrs M had invited them to Australia, all expenses paid for. I sat down with them and, although they had no interest in my programs because they were government sponsored courses for Australian citizens, they were quite happy to talk to me. I asked them why they were here and they sheepishly said that they had come on Mrs M's invitation. Would they send any students to us?

"On no" was the answer, "People in Uzbekistan don't have money to travel and certainly not to study overseas."

They weren't really sure why they were invited. They were quite amazed.

As far as I could see, Mrs M had lost all touch with reality. In fact, she showed many symptoms of schizophrenia. She couldn't see the big picture, but could get stuck on little details. She made many irrational decisions but was able to convince people around her that she was right. She was highly intelligent and very manipulative. Her mood swings were increasingly extreme and out of control. I started praying for her and myself. My main prayer for myself was to keep my heart clean and for her to be saved and to be taken to a psychiatrist for a diagnosis and medication.

When I went home at the end of every day, I shared some of these concerns with Jen but tried not to bring too much stress home. Jenny was still working through her own issues, trying to make sense of the last 6 years, so I kept all the weird news of what was happening at work to a minimum.

One Friday afternoon, I was sitting at my desk in our small staffroom. I was feeling quite content, as it had been a good week. The courses were running well and the students were happy to be studying with us. The other teachers had gone home for the weekend and I was tidying up a few last things before going home, too. The phone rang. I picked it up and heard Mrs M's voice:

"I want you to sack that sour woman."

"Excuse me? Who? What's going on?"

She was irate and wanted me to fire Geraldine because she had had enough of her. She was a sour grape and she had never liked her. I had to get rid of her. I protested and defended Geraldine for a while but there seemed to be no point. I told Mrs M that this was unlawful dismissal and that she could be taken to court. She didn't care; she didn't ever want to see Geraldine again. She hung up the phone. I sat there for a while, considering what to do. Geraldine was a good professional and a reliable employee. We had worked together since I started at this college about three and a half years ago. We had a good working relationship and friendship although we never socialized. I rang her and explained the situation and emphasized that I totally disagreed with Mrs M of course. She understood and told me that she would probably sue the college for unfair dismissal. She had to discuss this with her husband first. I went home with a heavy heart.

The next week Mrs M visited our building unexpectedly. She hardly ever came over so I was on edge. She had come with Sheila, the supervisor of the business program – an overdressed snotty woman with way too much make-up on and bright-red false nails. I was called into the tiny manager's office, which was usually empty, and Mrs M sat next to me. Sheila was sitting behind the desk and started. They had decided that she was now taking over the migrant programs and I would be working under her. Then as usual Sheila's mobile went off and she answered the call. Mrs M leaned over to me and whispered:

"If that Geraldine woman sues the college, I will make you responsible."

Sheila hung up the phone and continued babbling about how she was going to run my programs. I switched off and was thinking about Mrs M's threat. She would probably take me to court and somehow blame me for the unfair dismissal. The problem was that I had no money to defend myself while she could use the company's lawyer on company expense. This was not good. Then Mrs M took over and told me who in my staff were good teachers and who were not. She had walked past all the classrooms and in a split second had made the decisions by glancing through the glass doors. If a teacher happened to be standing up and talking to the students, they were good teachers. If the teacher happened to be sitting down in front of the class, they were lazy and incompetent. They should be active. The fact that the class might have been reading silently or doing a writing exercise didn't matter to her. I didn't argue because I now knew I was dealing with a totally irrational schizophrenic. There was no point.

This was all very stressful. These programs were my baby and I had worked hard to make them successful despite the lack of support from management and now I had to deal with this new supervisor who had no idea about migrants or English as a Second Language. Then I had a possible court case hanging over my head which would ruin me financially. It was so clear to me how mentally disturbed people wreak havoc in other people's lives. Why was I always in these situations? Why did I have to deal with psychopaths all the time? I felt so discouraged and exhausted from it all. I wished I could leave and move somewhere far away. This is all so unfair. At home things were finally going better and now I had to deal with this madness. I prayed incessantly for the Lord "to keep my heart with all diligence".

A few days later I was teaching my class and was pondering my future with this college. It looked so hopeless and I felt very burdened and stressed. I felt I had no options; I couldn't just walk out. I was trapped. My thinking was interrupted by a clear, loud voice from above:

"You are working for Me!"

I looked up although I was aware that the voice was in my head only. I knew it was the Lord and I knew what it meant. I had to focus on why I was there. I was doing His work with the migrants and He was my boss, not Mrs M or Sheila. I felt great relief. God would look after me despite all the chaos.

It was difficult to work with Sheila. She didn't have any understanding of what we were doing and made decisions about courses without consulting with me. She changed dates and informed the government department but neglected to inform me. The department then phoned me to ask what was going on. Why had we changed the starting dates? I apologized but told them that I was no longer in charge and that they had to contact Mrs M if they had any complaints. I then had to try and get in touch with Sheila who was never around and when I finally met with her in a coffee shop, she spent half her time on her mobile phone organizing her next golf game. I was furious while I was sitting there having to listen to her phone conversation, looking at her false eye lashes, fake red nails and arrogance and ignorance written all over her face. When she finally came off the phone, I complained about her making decisions without knowing about the history of the program, the contract with the government and without informing me. I tried to sound polite but firm. However, she was not willing to see she had done anything wrong and then waffled on about how busy she was. I interrupted her and told her I had to go back to work and left the coffee shop. Since then I never heard from Sheila again and I was left alone. Later on I was told that Sheila was relieved from her responsibility to supervise my programs because she was too busy.

In the meantime, Geraldine was taking the college to court for unfair dismissal and suing them for lost income and Mrs M told me that she would make me a third party and sue me for the cost of this court case. My only way out was to talk Geraldine out of taking the college to court. However, she was not prepared to do that and apologized to me for being caught in the middle. I was praying for this to blow over and started thinking about leaving. This 'dream job' had become way too stressful and I needed to get out. I discussed this with Jenny and she was happy for me to leave. She was working in a kindergarten as an assistant again and although she wasn't making much money, with some government assistance, we could probably get by. Jenny had been telling me for months that I looked terribly tired and had big black rings under my eyes. I kept saying that I was OK, but now I became aware that I was feeling really drained and worn out. I needed a break. I also had an idea for a business; I wanted to develop English teaching materials and sell them on my own website. One of the computer teachers at work was going to build the website for me.

On the weekend I wrote a letter of resignation and handed it in to Mrs M's secretary on Monday. That afternoon, Mrs M was on the phone telling me how sorry she was to see me go and asking me to reconsider. When I told my class of migrants that I was quitting, they were very upset. They told me that I was the best teacher they had had in Australia and that I treated them with respect.

"In the other college they treat us like children; you treat us like adults."

I thanked them for their compliments, but told them that the college was taking me to court and that I really needed to have a break. They decided to write a letter to Mrs M stating their feelings about me. They showed it to me the next day. It was the nicest letter I had ever read and they had all signed it. I am a loyal person but I was pushed too far and once I had made a decision I stuck with it. I felt greatly relieved.

We worked out the date of my leaving the college. I could actually take some holidays owed to me and leave in a fortnight. Because the college was in turmoil over other bad decisions that were made and was getting deeper and deeper in debt, there was no send-off party for me. The teachers said goodbye and thanked me for being such a good boss. The migrants said goodbye, some with tears in their eyes. They said they understood and wished me all the best. It was the greatest feeling walking out of that building for good.

A couple of months later, I received a letter from a solicitor. I was made a third party in the wrongful dismissal case and had to find a lawyer to defend myself. After some enquiries I found a Christian lawyer who was willing to help although he usually only handled big cases. He had an excellent reputation but cost $200 an hour. He said that this was expensive but he would keep the hours to a minimum and was almost sure this case would never go to court. Over the next couple of months, he corresponded with Mrs M's lawyer and realized that they were playing games. He asked me whether this woman knew what she was doing because the case didn't make any sense. Mrs M was trying to prove that I had had no authority to employ Geraldine and therefore was responsible for the dismissal. Since my job description clearly stated that recruitment of new teachers was my duty and I had been doing that for almost three years, the accusation was dropped and we never went to court. I knew that Mrs M was just doing it out of spite but it cost me $2,000 to defend myself against this false accusation. Although Geraldine had promised me to stop the court case, she went ahead with it without informing me. It was disappointing and especially when she received a pay-out from the college but never offered to pay some of my legal costs.

I never saw Mrs M again, but over the next years I heard that she had completely ruined the college. The Japanese management in Osaka finally fired her and sent the big boss's son to Australia to see if he could salvage the college which was now in huge debt. Many of the programs had been taken over by other colleges and there was only a very small remnant of English language students. Eventually they closed it down.

CHAPTER 12 Normality at home Nerang (8), Gold Coast, 1997- 1999

The next year and a half I stayed home and worked on writing and producing English language teaching materials. After the court case was over, I really enjoyed being at home and not having to deal with the stress of a mentally unstable boss. I started the day with getting the kids ready to go to school and doing the housework. I preferred to work in a well-organized and clean environment. Then I would spend the rest of the morning and early afternoon writing and submitting proposals to publishers. In the afternoon I picked up the kids from school and cooked dinner. Now Jenny was settled on her medication and feeling good most of the time, the house was peaceful and I started to relax for the first time in years. We were in a nice routine and were all enjoying family life. We did normal things as a normal family, relatively normal anyway. I realized one day that my neck had relaxed and I hadn't had a migraine in many months.

When you are dealing with severe mental illness, there are always unusual things to deal with because anti-depressants and anti-psychotic drugs have a lot of side-effects. For Jenny this meant for the first time in her life she was putting on weight. Over the next six months she had to change her wardrobe a few times. Luckily, there were a lot of second-hand clothing shops on the Gold Coast and it became a hobby for Jen to visit them. She had a knack for finding amazingly nice and almost new blouses and skirts, pants and shoes and anything else she wanted. It saved us thousands of dollars. I didn't realize how much weight she had gained until we were in a swimming pool one day and I saw her coming out of the water. In fact, I didn't recognise her at first with her wet hair stuck on her head. She was about double the size she was when she was ill. When we talked about it, she just calmly said that she would lose the weight. And amazingly she did in a few months. She just halved the size her meals and cut out all sweets. She didn't seem to find that hard at all.

With her constant need for change, she often surprised me by dying her hair. It was blond one day and red the next. Then she grew it and changed it to dark brown and then added streaks of various colors. Then it was cut short again. With her change of weight and clothing, I had the feeling I had a series of wives over the years. And I was not the only one. We had frequented the same shopping center for at least five years now. All the shop assistants knew us and we knew them. I was used to saying hello and they would nod or return with a greeting and an occasional chat. One day we went shopping. Jenny looked gorgeous. Her face shone happily and the clothes she was wearing showed off her great figure. I caught the eye of one of the female shop owners. She smiled at me and nodded. Then she looked at Jenny and her facial expression changed to one of disgust. She obviously didn't recognize her and probably thought that I was having an affair. I started to notice similar reactions from other people around me. I couldn't blame them.

At times the improvement seemed agonizingly slow. This is typical when you are in the middle of changes; things always change too slowly. You always want it to be over. This is obviously the way God teaches us patience. Overall, Jenny was coping quite well. We had made some new friends and started to have some kind of social life, though still limited. Jenny could never be out with people for too long and needed to return home to relax and have quiet around her. However, this was all very manageable.

The Lord kept working on me and continued to teach me, precept upon precept. One Sunday in church, I was convicted by the Holy Spirit of my involvement in Jenny's illness. I had always seen myself as a victim in the whole process of her becoming ill. I just happened to be there. That day the preacher was explaining the chain of command and the role of the husband in a Godly marriage and family. He is the head of the household under Christ followed by the wife and kids. It suddenly occurred to me that I had not fulfilled that role very well and was at least partly to blame for the fact that the devil had run riot in my family for so long. I usually took second place after Jenny and let her decide on all the spiritual issues. That was going to change now but first I felt burdened to apologize to her about my lack of leadership and protection. It was urgent so I asked her in the middle of the sermon to follow me outside the church. With tears in my eyes I apologized and asked for her forgiveness. Although she was somewhat surprised, she did immediately understand the issue and forgave me on the spot. We hugged and went back into the church to our seats.

Jenny was a woman of few words but when she spoke she often cut to the core of the issue. I was wondering what to do with my life. The materials I was writing were not selling and I couldn't find a publisher. Most publishers didn't even respond to a submission. I was expressing my frustration to Jenny one day and, as was usual now, she just listened. After a few minutes she asked me:

"What do you really want to do?"

This question took me by surprise because nobody had asked me that for ages. The answer I gave surprised me too:

"I want to do Bible study."

"OK, so go and do it."

It was that simple. I enrolled the next day and studied part-time for the next five months. It was wonderful.

For the next ten years Jenny was doing well despite an occasional lapse. When there was stress, she would suddenly slip back into depression. We would then have to adjust or change her medication and wait. It always takes at least a couple of weeks for anti-depressants and anti-psychotic drugs to take effect. With Jenny there was usually a quicker initial reaction and then a slow but steady improvement over many months. However, she also had some bad side-effects with a number of the drugs and they then had to be changed.

We did a lot of reading on natural health and discovered fish oil. We read that the omega 3 in fish oil could have a dramatic effect on mental illness, so we tried it. It took many months but the effect was indeed dramatic. Jenny became much clearer in her mind and more cheerful. The anti-psychotic medicine she had been taking for years numbed her brain and she had become quite passive and quiet. We could sit in the car for an hour and a half without her saying anything. The fish oil made her come alive a little more and her dry sense of humour returned. We also determined that an untreated post-natal depression was the most likely cause of all her troubles.

CHAPTER 13 Another irrational boss
Nerang (9), Gold Coast, 1999 - 2001

My new business wasn't working at all. I had put up a website but no orders came. I emailed a hundred different institutions all over the world but no response. After a year and a half of trying, money was very tight and I had to go back to work. Geraldine was working for a pleasant, small college in Surfers' Paradise, the tourist center of the Gold Coast, and had talked to the Director of Studies about me. I didn't really want to work for another language college, especially not a Japanese run college but I didn't have any choice and they were looking for a new teacher. I was introduced to the Director and she offered me a job after an informal chat. She said she knew enough about me and trusted Geraldine's recommendation. I could start on Monday.

Coming back to a staffroom was like coming home to a familiar place. I knew the kind of people, the books, the programs and the students, so it was easy to settle into this new job. I actually quite enjoyed being back in the classroom and it was a relief that there would be money in the bank at the end of every fortnight.

Since the Managing Director had left a month ago, the college was run by the director of studies. She was a very competent woman but doing two managerial jobs was too much. Also the admin staff, marketing manager and teachers didn't seem to get along. They didn't talk to each other apart from an awkward 'hello' or 'good morning'. I just did my job and, as usual, was friendly to everyone. After a few months we were told they had finally found a new Managing Director. It was a tough position to fill because there was relentless pressure from the Japanese mother company to increase profits. If a college made record profits one month, the next month the target was set even higher. It was a very demanding job.

The new MD, Mr Kieren Powell, was a tall skinny guy with a shaved head and bright blue eyes. He looked very pale and sickly and was full of nervous energy and I thought "there's something not quite right". We heard he had rung the Japanese manager for Australia three or four times a week to push his application and she had finally given in and given him the job. He was totally inexperienced in running a college and managing people and created confusion among staff right from the start. The Director of Studies often came out of the MD's office frazzled. She told us that he had no idea what he was doing but he wouldn't listen. He wanted changes and she didn't. It didn't take long before she resigned and we were without a Director.

Nobody including me wanted the job. I was the only one in the college who had the experience but I had no intention of complicating my life and working for another unstable boss. Rumors circulated that he had been fired from his previous teaching job because he had struck a Korean student in anger. When Kieren changed his computer to a laptop, he wanted all his emails, a couple of hundred of them, transferred from his old desktop to his laptop. He couldn't work out how to, so he hired a typist from an employment agency to retype all these emails. This took a couple of weeks. The temp was utterly confused why she was doing this, because as she told us most of these emails were of no use. After three weeks, and of course a couple of thousand dollars in wages, the temp was finished.

Kieren had been advertising for months for a new director to no avail. He gave up and instated his own wife as the Director. She was on leave from her job at another company and would be there for two months. She spent hours in Kieren's office and it became clear that he could not make a decision without consulting her first. She seemed quite competent and the college was at peace for a while. She created a buffer zone between Kieren and us.

After two months, however, Kieren's wife had to return to her job and he was left to his own devices. We noticed he spent a lot of time on the phone to her and every time a decision had to be made, however small, he had to ring her first. In the meantime his reputation had spread around the Gold Coast and it was hard to find teachers and impossible to find a new Director of Studies. Kieren was trying to do both jobs but things were not running very smoothly and we were losing students. At times we were down to under a hundred students and I could only imagine the pressure from Japan. Kieren's people skills, or rather lack thereof, didn't improve the situation. Everyone was on edge. I just did my job and watched the college deteriorate. I often had to laugh at his use of language in meetings. He seemed to be unable to pronounce certain words and was unaware of the errors he made. One of his favourite words was 'phenomena' but always came out as 'phenonema', even when it should have been the singular 'phenomenon' and 'academic' sometimes came out as 'epidemic'. He had also picked up on some trendy words such as 'prioritize' and 'guesstimate'. Sometimes it was hard not to laugh. One day he organized a friend of his who was a masseur to give us a neck and shoulder massage as a treat for our hard work. He kept referring to him as a 'masseuse'. I didn't know how to correct him politely so I didn't say anything.

With the lack of leadership the college continued on a downslide. New teachers didn't know where to find materials and were not told about the college's procedures. Processes became unclear and Kieren was often too busy or not around to make decisions. The number of student complaints increased dramatically and admin staff didn't know how to handle them. After a few months of this growing chaos, I decided to step in. I did really like this college and I thought that maybe God had put me there for this purpose. I also thought that because of my experience with mental illness, I was the best man to deal with Kieren. I talked with Jenny about it and as usual she was very supportive. The next day, I asked Kieren if I could apply for the director's position. He looked visibly relieved and said he had been waiting for my application but didn't want to push me. As he still had to go through the proper procedure with me, we set a date for an interview. I was excited and nervous at the same time.

The day of the interview arrived and we ended up in a tiny interview room upstairs rather than Kieren's office. He didn't want us to be disturbed. He had some sheets of white paper in front of him and a pen and started drawing a mind-map and explaining his vision for the college. He was quite hyper and talked non-stop for about forty-five minutes while madly scribbling notes on his mind-map which ended up covering three pages. He then handed me the unreadable scribbles as if they constituted some kind of invaluable document and told me that I was hired. He had not asked me one question and most of what he had told me made no sense. To some degree, I had anticipated a strange interview but this was much worse than I had expected. Driving home, I was somewhat bewildered but stuck with my decision to help "rescue" the college. There was a lot to learn, I would be in charge again and there would be a salary increase. I was put on six-month probation.

Things went much better than I expected. Kieren gave me the space to take charge of the college and he didn't interfere with the decisions I made. He got busy organizing a new computer network and started putting all admin and teaching resources on the new server. To improve communication between the teachers, admin and the marketers, we decided to have one representative of each department do a presentation about their job description and their duties. It opened the eyes of everyone as all now saw how busy the other staff members were and what they were trying to achieve. It became clear that we were all in this business together and that if we worked together we would all benefit because in the end we all wanted to keep our jobs. The college was turned around very rapidly and student numbers doubled in the next six months. Kieren was thrilled with my performance and cc-ed me an email to the managing director of another college praising my performance. He cut my probation period short by two months and gave me another raise.

Walking out of the office one day, he repeated that things were going very well and "that the gods must be with us". Maybe I should have kept my mouth shut but said that there was only one God and, yes, He was with us. He knew I was a Christian and he gave me a dirty look. A few days later he made the comment that all Buddhists think they are self-controlled, al Hindus are self-realized and all Christians self-righteous. This time I didn't say anything, but became aware that there was a spiritual warfare going on and I started praying for his salvation.

Kieren's hours became irregular and he appeared at odd times looking very distracted. On a number of occasions, he told me he had spent most of the night on his computer replying to emails or struggling with technical problems. He started wearing more and more black which contrasted strongly with his pale skin and made him look even more sickly. I tried to encourage him by reminding him that the college was doing well and that he could leave the daily running of the place with me. I even told him a few times that I enjoyed working for him because he gave me the space to be independent. His response was usually a cold distant stare which was an odd reaction.

Other issues emerged. One of the secretaries came to me one day because she was concerned about the Visa card statements. Kieren used the college credit card and in the last three months she had noticed more and more personal expenses on the statements. She had approached him about it but he had been evasive and told her that she was no longer allowed to open the Visa statements. They now had to go straight to his in-box, unopened. The expenses were running into the thousands of dollars. I told her to leave it with me.

Christmas was around the corner and a number of students and teachers would be going on holidays. This meant that the college would shrink temporarily and I was told to increase the number of students per class to twenty-two or more. This was against NEAS regulations. NEAS is the national body that oversees English language colleges in Australia. One of their strict rules is not to exceed eighteen students per class. So I was asked to go against the law and I refused. I showed Kieren the numbers of remaining students and teachers and calculations that showed we would not be losing any money. However, he didn't want to listen and pushed me to get it organized.

Then one day Kieren wanted to see me after classes but didn't say why. I got apprehensive when the time approached but kept my cool. We went upstairs to a classroom and he asked one of the secretaries to join us to take notes of what was said. He looked very stressed and started to tell me that he was not happy with my performance. He subsequently criticized me for the next hour and a half. I was told that my computer skills were inadequate, that my management style was pathetic and that I was unapproachable. He went on and on and was speaking in an irritable voice. I was absolutely flabbergasted. Where did all this come from? Just a few weeks ago he had praised my performance and now this. I just sat there and said nothing. I had no idea what to say to this uncontrollable barrage of negativity and thought there was no point in arguing with this irrational behavior. The secretary looked increasingly uncomfortable but kept taking notes. She told me later she couldn't believe what she heard and thought it was all his madness coming out. There was no truth in it and I shouldn't take it to heart. It was hard not to.

I spent the weekend in a confused daze. Jenny tried to encourage me and help me see the criticism was utterly irrational but I needed time to recover from this unexpected attack. It was good that Kieren would be on holidays for the next two weeks so I had time to think. I came up with a plan: I listed ten of Kieren's accusations on a worksheet and had choices under every statement from "I totally agree" to "I totally disagree". On Monday I called a short informal meeting for all staff, told everyone what had happened and asked them to fill out the questionnaire anonymously. I said that I would probably be fired but needed to know what they thought. The staff were infuriated by this attack on me and all questionnaires were back on my desk the same day. Except for one, they were all extremely positive about my management skills. Comments were added that I was the best Director they had ever worked for. I was strict but fair and they wanted me to stay. I was touched by the comments.

In addition to this, I talked to some of the teachers including Geraldine, and we decided to contact head office in Japan. We wrote an email to the manager of the Australian colleges whom we had met a few times. She seemed like a reasonable person. We expressed our concerns about Kieren's management of the college and the finances. We thought that if we mentioned money mismanagement, they would take this seriously. We were of course greatly aware of what happened last time we wrote to the Japanese management of the previous college.

Kieren now became simply known as K. Stories about K's reputation had spread around the Gold Coast and many of our teachers were leaving for other colleges. Most ended up at the local private university which had a magnificent campus and a director who was well-known for being a great boss. She supported the teachers and was very fair. The teachers from our college were called 'refugees' and K was now labeled 'the psychopath'. I was constantly recruiting new staff. Advertising, sifting through numerous resumes and interviewing took a lot of my time. Geraldine had also decided to leave when she was offered a job at the university language center. I sent in my CV and all my 'refugees' vouched for me. So it looked like I had somewhere to go when I left this job. It was clear to me that I couldn't stay. I had prayed about it for many months. I had asked the Lord to either change Kieren completely or remove him from the college. Neither of those had happened so I had to accept that it was my time to go.

When K came back from holidays, he was surprised to see that I was still there. He actually told me that he was amazed that I hadn't left. The same afternoon he called me into his office and asked me to close the door. He had received an email from Japan and was very disappointed that I had gone behind his back. I told him that we were very concerned about the college and his management and felt we had to do something. He looked very frightened but said that he couldn't trust me anymore. I didn't respond and we moved on to discussing the upcoming Christmas party. The relationship turned cold but I couldn't care less. I had done my very best to turn this college around and knew I had been successful in doing so. I was going to leave anyway: it was just a matter of deciding when exactly.

The Christmas party was reasonably pleasant. K gave a speech about how great the college was doing and made a point of thanking me personally for my hard work. K's wife was there and I couldn't help noticing how stressed she was. She used to be a fairly laid-back, calm person when she was the director of the college but now she had rings under her eyes and was constantly wringing her hands. She had a nervous tone in her voice and I really felt for her. If anyone, I could understand what she was going through with a husband who was mentally ill and spent most nights pacing the house. I desperately wanted to talk to her but this was not the right time or place and I prayed that the Lord would give me another opportunity at a later date. That never happened.

A few days later we had Christmas drinks again at the college. It was Friday afternoon after work and K was nowhere to be found. We all knew he was uncomfortable being with us, especially after I had given him my questionnaires. He knew the staff was behind me. We had had a few drinks when he arrived. He called me into his office and asked me if I had organized the larger classes for the Christmas period. I said that I hadn't because it didn't make sense as we were not losing money. He argued that it was not my decision to make and that I should follow his directions.

"But it is against NEAS regulations. I refuse to go against the law."

He kept insisting and I finally yelled back at him looking him straight in the eyes:

"Give me one good reason why I should do this? It doesn't make any sense!"

"I don't have to give you any reason. I am the managing director and I told you to change class sizes."

I walked out of his office and said loud enough so he could hear:

"I am sick of this bullshit."

I was quite aware that I was so outspoken because I had had a few drinks but I felt a great relief. It was an awesome experience to finally stand up for myself to an abusive boss. K was the third one and I had really had enough. I walked out of the building and drove home. I was euphoric.

Everybody was surprised to see me arrive back at work on Monday morning, but I was now defiant. This director's position was my job and I would decide when it was time to leave. K wanted to have a meeting with me on Wednesday; I had no idea what was going to happen now. Wednesday came but mid-afternoon I got a phone call from Jenny asking me if I could pick up the kids from school early because Mitchel was sick. I asked the secretary to apologize to K for having to postpone the meeting and left. The next day he was very annoyed about this because he had invited a lawyer to come all the way from Brisbane to join us. Brisbane was an hour by car and I hadn't shown up. That was expensive. When I asked him why, he didn't give me a straight answer and we rescheduled the meeting for early the next week.

When we sat down for the meeting, I was very curious what this was about. The lawyer looked somewhat uncomfortable as K started to dictate a list of demands, some of which were practically impossible and some of which could get me into trouble with the accreditation board. They would all be listed in a legal document that I had to sign. He wanted me to fulfill all these new duties and if not, there would be consequences. The whole court case with Mrs M flashed before my eyes and I was not going to be sued again by some nutcase who had a company behind him to pay his legal expenses.

"I quit!"

K looked stunned and said:

"Excuse me?"

"I said I quit."

K didn't know what to say. I got up, said goodbye to the lawyer and left the meeting. My stomach was nervously vibrating but I was ecstatic and proud of myself. I was smiling while I walked to my desk.

The next day we worked out the details of my leaving. My time was cut short by taking up some holidays that were owed. The staff was very upset but understood that I had had enough, especially when I told them what stunt K had pulled this time. To my surprise, K agreed to having a farewell party at the college and even more surprisingly the college had contributed to a farewell present for me. K then proceeded to give a speech thanking me for all the hard work in turning this college around and wishing me all the best in the future. He actually had tears in his eyes. He would write me a good reference if I needed one. I decided that would probably not be a good thing considering his reputation. Looking into his eyes, I saw how lost he was and genuinely hoped he would find his way to a good psychiatrist and be put on medication. God knew that I had prayed for him regularly for many months. However, I had done more than my best to help him and I needed to save myself and keep my sanity.

CHAPTER 14 Last days in Australia Nerang (10), Gold Coast, 2001

"Yes, I know what you have been through with that crazy Kieren. I have heard all the stories and all your 'refugees' here vouch for you so I don't need to interview you. You have the job."

The Director of Studies at Bond University English Language Institute came straight to the point. I liked that. She looked like a typical academic, somewhat cool and lacking a sense of humour but I had heard very positive reports about her from my previous employees and they said she was very 'sane'. That was all that mattered to me. I could start work on Monday.

It was like another home-coming. I was working in a cramped staffroom with a lot of my old colleagues and I was back in the classroom. My days became routine very soon and I thoroughly enjoyed the job. The classes had a nice mix of nationalities which always made for more interesting lessons and discussions. The campus consisted of a number of old-style, sandstone clad buildings arranged around a lake on one side and well-kept sloping gardens through the middle bordered by broad staircases. It was a pleasure to walk to class at the other end of the campus and to go and buy some lunch and sit at the lake. I started to relax and enjoy life again for the first time in many years.

In the meantime, Jenny had made her own changes to her life. She had left the kindergarten and decided to do a course in diversional therapy. She had met a Christian lady who worked in an old people's home and had asked her to come and do some voluntary work. She really enjoyed working with elderly people and decided to do a course to become a qualified diversional therapist. Knowing that Jenny always needs changes, I encouraged her. She was very settled and although studying for the first time in many years was quite a challenge, she seemed to be coping fine. The study made her mind more active and the new work seemed to make her determined to succeed.

Life was so normal. In the olden days that would have bored me to death. I was not the conventional type and very little in my life had been conventional. Meeting Jenny at Central Station in Amsterdam was a surprise to start with and everything after that had been unpredictable. That's the way I used to like it but after so many years of weird behavior and difficulties, I was ecstatic about the normality in my life. Things were predictable now but I knew somewhere in the back of my mind that that wouldn't last. Restlessness grew in my spirit and I felt a need to make changes especially to be financially more relaxed so I didn't have to watch every cent we spent.

Mental illness needs constant management. There may be long periods where everything is going well and the patient is very settled and functional. Then suddenly the medication is not as effective as it used to be and either the dosage needs to be adjusted or the medication, usually one of the pills only, needs to be changed. These periods of peace for Jenny would usually last for about three years before there would be a relapse and we needed to reassess her cognitive functions with the psychiatrist. Some psychiatrists confirmed to me that most of their patients show these cycles. When this happened the first time, I was devastated and thought we were starting all over again. But when Jenny recovered within a month and seemed to be functioning even better than before, I accepted that this was something we had to expect and get used to. The study had taken its toll and as I had learnt stress was the main trigger for another episode. Jenny started to withdraw and the expression on her face showed a certain gloom.

Well, it's another relapse and the first time that I have decided to take control of my illness as best I can with the help of Jesus Christ in my life and times of constant prayer to guide me through. I now have a hold on the things happening to me yet again. The voices are God's, my conscious and subconscious thoughts, other people's conscious and subconscious thoughts and in the beginning when my mind was not healed by the Lord I was tormented with a barrage of both spiritual and mortal voices and thoughts. Having been through my experience there is no doubt in my mind that Satan's dark and evil forces do exist. Just as the beautiful light and life of Christ is so real in my awareness, made possible by Christ in me, I cannot begin to describe the truth as I have lived it.

God has healed me by faith over and over again just as He promises. This last stage of healing was because I didn't want to have to begin taking the anti-psychotic drug again as this would create another zombie-like effect and would make me gain weight again, probably make me twice the normal size. Instead I chose to deal with my relapse totally by prayer, and then my mind began to unravel like a ball of string.

First for His way to reach me was to deal with the subconscious thoughts and past beliefs I had. Whether these thoughts were real or not, my understanding during that time meant that God used these to start healing me and was then be able to show that even though I was unwell, he could still reach me and eventually heal that part of me. He is truly the physician that the Bible promises.

Forgiveness and repentance were the keys to healing and well-being, all done in the name of Jesus Christ, and finally acceptance that he did in fact die on the cross for my sins and therefore I had no reason to carry anything anymore.

It was incredible; because of the nature of who I am I believed I had to go through a process of healing. Clearly any other Christian could quite easily believe that it was all done on the cross for us, accepted Christ and recognized what he had done on the cross for us and be done with it all and moved on from there. Not me however, I was stubborn. I obviously thought that I had to have a hand in it or maybe God wanted it this way so that my dream of being destined to have a great impact on the world in the name of Jesus would come to fruition.

During this relapse I was in prayer for most of the time I was awake. No little thing was overlooked, from making coffee or tea and how much to drink was crucial. I prayed constantly for discernment of voices. I only wanted to respond to the voice of God. It was however vitally important that I heard the other voices as well. If I was to respond to God, I had to listen to the other voices. I needed for example to hear what I believed about myself subconsciously so that I could forgive or repent when necessary.

It was at this time that the lord showed me how the voices worked. Other people's conscious/subconscious thoughts enter and leave everybody's mind and affect other people. Most people are not aware of it. But because of the nature of myself I was always confused about which voice was the voice of God.

Therefore whenever I heard the voice of God now, I prayed in the name of Jesus Christ who died on the cross for my sins and covered myself with the blood of Christ, and then and then only did I trust that the voice was from God.

We had believed in a guru who said he was the incarnation of Christ and since we studied the Bible and discovered that he was a fraud, it has always been a problem in the past for me to fully embrace my Christianity.

I had to find a way around this problem and I believe that I did because no one can copy Christ's death and resurrection.

My battles of the past were purely spiritual and it took a good 20 years to finally come to grips with it all. I realized that my mind had been so twisted and confused about what I believed on the surface and what I believed subconsciously. Now I could get through my day and function relatively normally. However, as soon as I became in any way spiritual I couldn't cope. I refused to believe that my only choice was to be a zombie on medication or spiritually screwed up and unstable.

For some reason God chose now to heal me His way. I had tried to deal with this before in much the same way but without success.

Once I had repented for all of the things that I had believed in the past and forgiveness was underway, everything started to calm down. No longer did I have to pray non-stop throughout the day and luckily it was just about time to return to work.

After a year the course was completed and Jenny became a certified Diversional Therapist. She also had a year's experience under her belt but the place where she was working didn't have any paid positions available so she decided to look for paid work elsewhere. It didn't take her long to find a full-time position as an activity officer with dementia patients in an aged care facility. We thought that would be perfect because she understood mental problems so well now and she was very patient. On the first day of her new job, Jenny was excited and quite nervous. She had visited the facility and had met the older people she would be working with. Her immediate boss was on holidays so she would meet her later. The first weeks went well. She followed the routine of gathering the people and doing activities as well as possible. Many of the patients were not really capable of following instructions anymore and sometimes they just ended up chatting. The elderly loved talking about their past and often relived it so vividly that Jen just sat and listened to their stories.

We had bought a little chiwawa that was shown on TV on an RSPCA show. He was a sweet, easy-going dog and the kids of course loved him. Jenny had decided to take him to work as she thought the old people would love to have a pet around. She asked for permission and took the dog to work on the first day her supervisor came back from holidays. She walked the dog into hall and ran into her boss who put her briefcase down to shake Jenny's hand. While they were getting to know each other, the dog was sniffing the briefcase. To Jenny's horror, he decided to lift his leg and pee on the briefcase. She apologized profusely but her boss just said:

"Don't worry; he probably just smelled my dog."

The dog was a great success. The old people all wanted to hold him and occasionally one decided to kidnap him and hide with him in the toilet, hoping Jen would go home without him.

My work was interesting. I loved having Brazilians, Europeans and an occasional Arab in my class as well as the usual Asians. I was teaching a pre-intermediate level which meant that students were able to have basic conversations and write basic emails but not more than that. It was the inter-cultural communication that made the lessons interesting. Brazilians were so outgoing and free whereas Asians especially the Japanese were very inhibited. I decided to ask the students to give short presentations about their countries and culture so they could learn from each other and by understanding each other better become more tolerant and accepting of their differences. One of the Brazilian students was happy to start and do her presentation the next day. She told us about the social life and relaxed lifestyle in Brazil. She wanted to impress on us how important the carnivals were so she had brought a tape of Brazilian music and asked if she could play some. I agreed of course so she put the tape in the recorder and pushed play.

"This is how we dance in my country."

She started swaying her arms and swinging her hips. She was wearing a fairly skimpy top and mini-skirt and I looked around to see how the Asians and Europeans would react. They looked quite embarrassed and uncomfortable. The presenter seemed oblivious of the class's reaction and danced to her heart's content. She suddenly stopped and we all clapped.

The presentation was only just finished when there was a knock on the door. One of the admin staff brought a new student to join the class. He was a big guy from the United Arab Emirates, 6 foot 5 like me but double my size. He shook my hand and introduced himself as Abdullah. I welcomed him into the class and told him what we were doing. He immediately volunteered to speak about his country and was ready to start. Although I appreciated his enthusiasm, I suggested he prepared himself and do it the next day. He was fine with that.

The next day came and Abdullah was prepared. He told us about the UAE, a small Arab country bordering Saudi Arabia. Oil had been discovered in the 50s and the country had become very wealthy. Everybody drove 4-wheel drives and housing and education for the local Arabs, the Emiratis, was free. Abdullah talked with enthusiasm about the desert, camping and the cities, Dubai and Abu Dhabi. Everyone was engrossed because we had never heard such positive talk about the Middle East. As I usually did at the end of these presentations, I asked him about work for English teachers and he told me there was a lot of work because the country was bilingual. When I heard him use the word 'bilingual', I realized how good his English had been through the whole presentation. He had hardly made any mistakes and seemed quite fluent. He continued to tell us that everybody at high school had to learn English and colleges and universities were all in English. Students would do IT or Business courses in English and therefore had to continue learning English to improve. I was sorry to have to stop the presentation but after half an hour I felt I needed to go on with other things. I congratulated him on being such a good ambassador for his country and asked the students to open their textbooks. The rest of the morning I taught on automatic pilot. I was very distracted after Abdullah's talk and couldn't focus on what we were doing in class.

When I got home that afternoon, I told Jenny about Abdullah and the UAE. She listened intently and said

"Let's go!"

I looked at her in amazement.

"That's not really what I meant. I don't want to live in a Muslim country. I can't imagine what that would be like."

Again she said: "Let's go. We've had enough of Australia. We are going nowhere here. The money you make is only just enough to live.

We can never do anything. We haven't had a holiday in years. Let's go to the UAE. Just pray about it and have a look online at the website of that college and see what happens."

After some discussion, I agreed to at least check it out and ask the Lord if that was what He wanted for us. However, before I sat down to pray, I already knew that Jen was right and that we were going to move to the Middle East.

The next day Abdullah was not in my class. When I asked administration what had happened to him, they told me that it had been a mistake. Abdullah should have been sent to an upper-intermediate class and not my pre-intermediate. That was not a surprise to me but had the Lord just put him in my class for the day to tell me about the UAE so we could go there? Deep inside I felt this was the case. I decided to make sure to take it seriously and apply for work online that night.

The Higher Colleges of Technology in the UAE are government-run colleges in every city in the country. Their website was very well organized. I read the information and applied online, which took a couple of hours. After I had finished, I felt I needed to relax a bit and played a game of solitaire. The game flowed so easily, I could move cards into the right places at high speed. And then out of the blue, the Holy Spirit came upon me. I wasn't even thinking about the Lord; in fact He was furthest from my mind but obviously I was on His mind. The game kept moving fast and I heard His voice:

"This is how it is going to work; everything will fall into place."

I knew that it related to our move to the UAE and that I didn't have to worry. Two issues had kept me concerned about moving. One was Jenny's healthcare. Were we going to find a good psychiatrist in the UAE? I had no idea what the situation was like over there. Would we be able to find the medicine she needed to stay stable? And secondly will we be able to sell the house? Times were tough and nobody was buying real estate. However, the few words God spoke that night set my mind at ease. I now knew I had to move in faith.

My colleagues suggested I talk to Douglas. He was a Canadian teacher who had lived in the UAE and in fact had worked for the Higher Colleges of Technology for ten years. Doug was very generous with his time and told me about the HCT and the UAE at every break time. He loved the place and so did his kids. We spent hours together and I built up a detailed picture of what life was going to be like. At night Jen and the kids would listen to all the stories. Initially the children were quite resistant to leaving behind everything they were familiar with and by then I had learnt not to force things. So I waited and prayed. I asked the Lord for harmony, for one mind, about the move and one day after weeks of deliberation both children came to us and said that they were ok to go. Mitchel was about to turn 13 and Chantelle was 10 and both were highly intelligent. They just needed time to get used to the idea.

Like the Lord told me during the card game everything fell into place. My application went through the various stages and was accepted. I had a nerve-racking hour-long video interview with a panel of four supervisors which went very well. I was 'in the pool' and any college around the country was able to offer me a position if my qualifications and experience suited their needs. So, the waiting started. However, there was plenty to do. We sold the house in record time and started packing and storing our belongings.

The last night in the house we slept on mattresses so the next morning we just had to pick up a few things including the TV and leave. We had booked a cabin in a caravan park for the last three to six weeks before we would fly out. It was risky but we were promised it shouldn't take any longer. Mitchel and Chantelle were watching TV while Jen and I were packing up the last things.

"Dad, there is something wrong with the TV. Every channel has the same picture."

I looked at the screen and noticed two sky-scrapers in a city I didn't immediately recognize. We flicked through the channels but the picture didn't change. Then, suddenly, we saw an airplane fly straight into one of the buildings.

"Oh, my God. What's that?"

I first thought it was an accident and wondered if the pilot had been drunk or asleep.

While the full story of 9/11 unfolded in the next couple of days, we became concerned how this would affect our move to the Middle East. Would it be cancelled? Would governments around the globe call all their people back home from the Middle East? Would a war break out? There were so many questions and we knew we just had to be patient and wait to see how the situation would develop. We were now stuck in a small cabin and the house was no longer ours. We couldn't go back. So, we prayed and believed that God would continue to make this an easy transition. In the meantime, we hadn't heard anything from the HCT, there still wasn't an actual job offer on the table. We carried on as normal. The children were still going to school and I still had to go to work. Jenny had given up her job and was organizing our finances and other effects so we would be ready to jump on a plane as soon as we got the call. Weeks went by in an almost eerie silence and then the phone rang.

"Good afternoon. My name is Marie Daymon. I am a supervisor at the Ras Al Khaimah Women's College. Is this a good time to talk or shall I call back later?"

Good or not, I couldn't wait any longer. I walked into the tiny bedroom and sat on the bed. Marie was not in a hurry. She took her time to explain details of the job, the college and the town. Jenny had joined me on the bed and was trying to pick up parts of the conversation. I repeated some of the information Marie gave me for Jenny's benefit.

"I am sorry I have to ask you this but are you by any chance Jewish? Your name could very well be so."

I replied that I wasn't and that I was a born-again Christian. Marie responded enthusiastically:

"Oh great, so am I".

She continued to tell me about the little church they ran and that they would be thrilled to have us there. I also wanted to know what the effect of 9/11 had been in the UAE. She reassured me that nothing had changed and that everything had continued as usual. If anything, the students felt sorry for the American teachers and some had apologised on behalf of all Arabs. After about forty-five minutes, Marie wanted to know if I was interested in the job. I asked her if she needed an answer immediately. Jenny looked at me intently and nodded her head. Her lips said:

"Take it. Take it."

And so we decided on the spot to accept the offer.

When exactly I was going to start was still unclear. The semester had started at the end of August and it was now the beginning of October. Marie had one teacher who wanted to leave as soon as possible but it all depended on how long it would take to get my security check finalized. That could take weeks or even months. Not really what we wanted to hear. We waited. These must have been the slowest weeks of my life and the silence from the UAE was deafening. I kept thinking "No news is good news" but after three weeks couldn't wait any longer and emailed them. Then in the middle of the night, the phone rang. We were fast asleep and the ring tone was nicely embedded into my dream. It took me a while to come to my senses and realise it was the telephone. I stumbled out of bed and tripping over bags and boxes, finally made it to the phone. It stopped ringing and so did my heart for a second. Thank God, I had signed up for an automatic answering service. I checked my messages and yes it was the HCT:

Mr Zimmermann, my name is Libby Walker and I am the Human Resource officer at the Ras Al Khaimah Colleges. I am afraid there has been a change of plans. In consultation with the supervisor at the Women's college, we have decided to..."

And that's where the message ended. I was horrified. What now? Decided to what? Oh God, I need to know. Why didn't that stupid answering service have more time for messages? My major fear was that they had decided that they didn't need me after all and we were stuck in a tiny, smelly cabin for another so many months while we would try and find a house and start over. I tried the redial service because I had no phone number. The phone rang and rang but nobody picked up. I realized it was 6 PM in the UAE and the HR person probably made the phone call and went home. All I could do was sent another email and hope I would have a response by the next afternoon. The 6 hour time difference was unbearable. It took me a long time to get back to sleep.

The next day Marie rang and apologized for the call in the middle of the night. My security clearance had come through and they had decided that they wanted me to come as soon as possible. If we were ready, they would courier the contract and the tickets that same day or early the next morning.

"Oh thank God. That's great news. Yes, we are ready. The sooner, the better actually."

"OK good, and don't worry about faxing the contract back to us. Just bring it with you. You should be here within a week or less."

CHAPTER 15 To the United Arab Emirates

Ras Al Khaimah, UAE, 2001

We flew out with Cathay Pacific at the beginning of November. There were TV screens in the back of every seat and with the endless supply of soft drinks, the kids thought they were in heaven. We had a stopover in Hong Kong and stayed the night in a beautiful 5-star hotel near the airport. Now Jen and I thought we were in heaven. We had a long sleep, a sauna and a lovely meal and everything was paid for. When we arrived in Dubai, a small bus took us to Ras Al Khaimah, to the newly opened Hilton Hotel. It was late at night and we just crashed. The next morning I was taken to the college to meet the director. He kept it very short, welcomed me and wished me all the best. The Human Resources lady gave me $750 for food and said my furniture allowance of $15,000 would be there in the afternoon. Having been given cash on the first day and staying in the Hilton for a week was a wonderful change from the life of scarcity we had been living for so long in Australia. Everything was as Doug had told me and because there were no real surprises, none of us felt any culture shock. We just enjoyed every minute of settling in to RAK and its community. It was a very friendly place. Many expats would come to my desk at work and offer help and some even rang us to introduce themselves and welcome us to town. Jenny was thriving. This was what she loved to do: buying new furniture and decorations for the house. They had given us a beautiful double-storey house in a complex with about 35 houses, a gym and a 25 meter swimming pool. Our house looked out over the inlet from the Gulf into town, so the view was great and in every other country this would be prime real estate.

The children made friends very quickly and quite a few of them lived in the complex, so they were also happy. In the first week, we all four went to the college to get a tour and have lunch. When we walked into the canteen, it struck me how culturally different we were. There were approximately three to four hundred Emirati girls in black robes and head scarves in the canteen and many looked at us when we entered. Mitchel was wearing a bright red t-shirt and board shorts, Chantelle a bright pink dress, Jenny a yellow top and green skirt and I wore a light blue shirt and bright blue tie. Some of the girls just smiled and welcomed us. I didn't know at the time that everybody was expecting the new teacher and his family and many even knew my kids' names.

We met Marie, my supervisor, that afternoon. She was the opposite body-type to me, short and chubby, but she demanded a hug to welcome me. My 6 foot 5 frame had to bend down to accommodate her. She had the most open smile and face I had ever seen. There was nothing hidden and she made it clear to me very quickly that "what you see is what you get." I took an immediate liking to her. She would take us to church that weekend.

Jen and I were aware that we had to start looking for a psychiatrist fairly soon because we didn't know whether it was a complicated process or not to get the medicine. We had found out that the meds were available before we arrived but didn't know how to get them. After some inquiries we found there was a good psychiatrist in Dubai and we made an appointment. He was an older man with a very gentle, pleasant manner. He explained the process of getting medicines through the government health system and that there was a good psychiatrist in Ras Al Khaimah so that we didn't have to come to Dubai every month. You could only get meds for a month at a time, which was exactly the same as in Australia. We organized to get a health care card and Jenny visited the psychiatrist, Dr Talaat, for the first time. I had to go to work but was anxious to hear what he was like when I got home. He was going to be a key person in our happiness in the UAE, so it was important that Jenny got on with him and they understood each other. To my great relief, they immediately clicked. Jenny thought he was an interesting man with a good sense of humour. He was Egyptian in origin but had worked in the UAE for many years. He had in fact set up psychiatry in the country. On top of all that he was a Christian as well. What a blessing!

I met Dr. Talaat early on in the UAE. He was a rather small but funny man with a great sense of humor which didn't go astray. He loved to talk but also had a great propensity to listen well. I instantly bonded with him. He always seemed to know exactly where I was at and what was to come next. Initially he dealt with my existing medications and symptoms until gradually he guided me into more appropriate medications for the particular symptoms I presented until finally he changed the original diagnosis when I was admitted to hospital on the Gold Coast. I went from depressive/schizophrenic to depressive/bipolar disorder, quite a change indeed. He explained was that it was quite common for symptoms to change. Anyway, the change of medication changed my temperament entirely and I had never felt better in my life. I was no longer sluggish and zombie-like. I was more attentive and involved. My emotions began to come alive once again. I could feel the love of my family around me once more and reciprocate. I was totally in love with being alive. There was no way that I would go back to my zombie existence, even though it did give me some semblance of order and peace.

Dr. Talaat made me believe that I could be a normal part of life and that I wasn't a misfit. I could hold down a job without these heavy sedatives and interact normally with people once more. Initially I wasn't sure. My emotions were all over the place but after a while they settled. People had to get used to me a bit but after a while I started to develop a little more of what I used to be like before I became ill.

Dr Talaat was happy with my progress. My visits with him were always very positive. He is a Christian and constantly reminded me to continue my prayer life and thank the Lord for all of the goodness He provides. Each visit over the years became very uplifting for both of us, him needing prayer for his work at the hospital and me needing further help with adjustments to my medication. We always parted, lifted in spirit and cheerful that the days ahead would be light for both of us.

Dr Talaat diagnosed what he called 'a symptom shift' and Jenny came alive as she came off the numbing anti-psychotic drug she had been on for the last ten years. Her emotions fluctuated for a couple of weeks but we decided to ride it out. Her emotions stabilized and she started to enjoy life with new gusto. I hadn't seen her like this since the early days of our relationship. I was very grateful to the doctor and thanked the Lord for him every day.

It didn't take long before Jenny was offered work in the kindergarten of the English-speaking school where the kids attended. She started work but within a few weeks, the supervisor of the ESL department came and talked to her. She said:

"Sorry, Jenny, but I happen to notice that you have experience teaching English as a Second Language and I need another teacher in Primary. Would you be willing to teach there?"

Jenny was thrilled to do that and, with the permission of management, changed jobs the next day. The supervisor was also a Christian.

I decided to read scripture and pray once in the morning and then just get on with what I had to do. My prayer was always for God to direct and guide me throughout the day and I would finish with "not my will but Your will be done, Lord."

Sure enough all through the day I would feel His presence. Even when I had to say something if it was the wrong thing to say no one would even hear me speaking. On the other hand, if I had to speak and God was with me I would feel this incredible urge to want to speak up.

I went to work every day but felt decidedly unwell, mentally. I could cope at home but at school, teaching a class of year one primary school children was to say the least very challenging.

Finally I went back to Dr Talaat and asked for something to help me, but not that heavy anti-psychotic medication that had kept me completely drugged for 10 years. It had given me much relief from the tormented life I had been leading; however my feelings and all emotional responses were totally quashed leaving me to be zombie like both day and night.

Dr Talaat prescribed another fairly heavy drug but I only needed small doses of it, 1mg twice daily. I continued taking three other meds: one anti-depressant and two mood-stabilizers. It took a week and a half and I started to feel more in control again.

The end of the first semester arrived and we had our first two-week holiday. It was January and the weather is beautiful at that time of year: sunny and around 25 degrees centigrade. We were invited to go camping with a Christian family that lived a few doors up from us and so we bought some camping gear. Yet another Christian colleague was kind enough to lend us her small 4 by 4. We couldn't believe that the Lord was surrounding us with so many Christians, the last thing we expected in a Muslim country. We packed the car and started on the journey to Oman. Leaving Ras Al Khaimah, we drove through the desert. On the left were the bare, rocky mountains that displayed different shades of red and brown in the sunlight. I looked at Jenny sitting next to me and noticed that she had a contented smile on her face. She looked so at peace.

FAQs for carers

What do I do when I noticed "there is something not quite right" with one of my loved ones or friends?

This is the toughest question to answer. If you find that someone close is showing strange symptoms or behavior or actually tells you that they are depressed, they really need to see a psychiatrist. To find one, ask your local doctor. The tricky part is to convince the person to go and see a psychiatrist. You will most definitely be confronted with a lot of resistance. Here are some points to consider and explain to the person:

- Mental illness, whether it is depression, bi-polar disorder or schizophrenia, is a chemical issue with your brain. Despite all the complex thoughts and feelings related to all these illnesses, they are in the end just a physical problem and can be treated with medication, the same way you would treat any other physical disease. Would you keep ignoring it if you had a heart disease, diabetes or cancer?
- Initially, one of the most sensitive issues is that the person is worried everybody, or even anybody, is going to find out that they are seeing a psychiatrist. Promise to keep it quiet and make sure to tell no one. If you want the person to trust you, you must make sure not to break the trust. You will often find later that they relax about this issue and they themselves start telling people around them about their treatment.
- Take your relative or friend to his/her first appointment, partly to support them but also to make sure they don't change their mind at the last minute.

What if the person refuses to go or is too disconnected with reality to make any decision?

When someone is seriously mentally ill and incapable of making a rational decision, you will have to make it for them. It is not a matter for discussion. For example, a schizophrenic may be extremely manipulative and will promise they will get the problem under control or try to convince you it is not a problem. At some stage, you must act as a carer and take them to a psychiatric ward or a psychiatrist.

What is the difference between a psychiatrist/psychiatry and a psychologist/psychology?

A psychiatrist is a medically trained doctor who is specialized in mental illness. They will diagnose the illness and prescribe medication. A psychologist is a trained in various kinds of psycho-analysis. They will try to solve problems through discussion.

Can psychology help?

Since mental illness is a physical illness, psychology won't help. Mentally ill patients can talk for hours about their inner feelings and problems they have had but nothing is resolved because the brain is not in a state to actually process and release the feelings. Once the brain is settled on medication and the patient is more functional and can have a rational discussion, psychology may be helpful in sorting out some personal problems. However, I highly recommend for Christians to find a good biblically based counselor, since Godly counsel is based on divine truth about who we are, whereas most psychological counseling is based on self.

Is mental illness a spiritual issue?

Most likely, since every problem has a spiritual aspect to it. However, it is highly recommended to start with

1. The physical: find a good psychiatrist to diagnose the person and get the patient settled on medication. Then they will be much easier to handle because their mind will function more rationally.
2. When the person is settled, find a good Christian counselor.

Are mentally ill people possessed by evil spirits?

Although a mentally ill patient may very well be possessed, it is highly recommended not to focus on it too much. It may freak out an already very vulnerable person. The last thing they need is being told they are possessed by an evil spirit.

Jesus set some very disturbed people free from evil spirits and they were healed instantly. Can we as Christians do this?

If it is led by the Holy Spirit, I have no doubt this is possible. However, I have never seen it myself. I have seen some Christian screaming and threatening poor mentally ill patients trying to free them from evil spirits. All that happened was that the patients became extremely upset and in fact were worse off for the experience. On the other hand, if a patient continuously feeds his or her own mind with scripture and prays, eventually evil spirits will not be able to withstand the light of Christ and will have to leave.

Useful references

A list of symptoms at www.sane.org[1]
http://www.sane.org/information/factsheets-podcasts/462-something-is-not-quite-right-checklist

---

1. http://www.sane.org

In various languages

http://www.sane.org/information/factsheets-podcasts/213-somethings-not-quite-right-translations[1]

1. http://www.sane.org/information/factsheets-podcasts/213-somethings-not-quite-right-translations

List of factsheets

http://www.sane.org/information/factsheets-podcasts[1]

124

---

1. http://www.sane.org/information/factsheets-podcasts

A book on brain research and natural medicines

Jean Carper, Your Miracle Brain: Maximize Your Brainpower, Boost Your Memory, Lift Your Mood, Improve Your IQ and Creativity, Prevent and Reverse Mental Aging

Coping with depression from a Christian viewpoint

Tan, S. Y., & Ortberg, J. (2004). *Coping with depression*. Baker Books.

9 798223 202561